Rafaella Maria Monteiro Sampaio
Francisco José M. Pinto
Débora Sâmara G. Dantas

Collective Health

Rafaella Maria Monteiro Sampaio
Francisco José M. Pinto
Débora Sâmara G. Dantas

Collective Health

Epidemiological approaches in evidence

ScienciaScripts

Imprint
Any brand names and product names mentioned in this book are subject to trademark, brand or patent protection and are trademarks or registered trademarks of their respective holders. The use of brand names, product names, common names, trade names, product descriptions etc. even without a particular marking in this work is in no way to be construed to mean that such names may be regarded as unrestricted in respect of trademark and brand protection legislation and could thus be used by anyone.

Cover image: www.ingimage.com

This book is a translation from the original published under ISBN 978-3-330-76277-0.

Publisher:
Sciencia Scripts
is a trademark of
Dodo Books Indian Ocean Ltd. and OmniScriptum S.R.L publishing group

120 High Road, East Finchley, London, N2 9ED, United Kingdom
Str. Armeneasca 28/1, office 1, Chisinau MD-2012, Republic of Moldova, Europe
Managing Directors: Ieva Konstantinova, Victoria Ursu
info@omniscriptum.com

Printed at: see last page
ISBN: 978-620-8-39142-3

AUTHORS / ORGANISERS

Rafaella Maria Monteiro Sampaio

Nutritionist. PhD student in Collective Health (UECE). Master in Public Health (UECE). Lecturer in Nutrition at the University of Fortaleza (UNIFOR) and the Estácio do Ceará University Centre.

Francisco José Maia Pinto

Statistician and Mathematician. Post-Doctorate in Collective Health (USP). PhD in Institute of Social Medicine (UFRJ). Master of Science in Production Engineering (UFRJ). Adjunct Professor at the State University of Ceará.

Débora Sâmara Guimarães Dantas

Nurse. PhD student in Collective Health (UECE). Master in Collective Health (UECE). Specialist in Health Systems and Services Management (ESP-CE). Specialist in Family Health (UFC). Specialist in Obstetric Nursing (ESP-CE).

AUTHORS / COLLABORATORS

Ana Maria Peixoto Cabral Maia
Physiotherapist. Specialist in Epidemiology and Health Surveillance (UFC).

Carlos Robson Bezerra de Medeiros
Statistician. Master in Maths (UFC). Specialist in Statistics (UFC). Lecturer at the Federal University of Ceará (UFC).

Dandhara Kathleen Monteiro Vaz
Biomedicine student at the Unichristus University Centre.

Daniele Silva de Oliveira
Nursing student at the Faculdade Integrada da Grande Fortaleza (FGF).

Elanny Cristina Pascôa Candeira
Physiotherapist. Resident in Collective Health at the Ceará School of Public Health (ESP).

Fiama Kécia Silveira Teófilo
Nurse. Master's student in Collective Health at the State University of Ceará.

Francisca Cláudia Monteiro Almeida
Nurse. Master in Public Health (UECE). Specialist in Family Health (ESP). Specialist in Labour Nursing (UECE). Nurse in the Family Health Strategy in the municipality of Fortaleza - CE.

Francisco Regis da Silva
Nutritionist. Master's student in Collective Health (UECE). Master's student in Agroindustrial Systems (UFCG). Specialising in Public Health (ESP-CE).

Geziel dos Santos de Sousa
PhD in Collective Health. Master in Public Health (UFC). Full degree in Geography (UECE) and BA in Geography (UECE). Professor at Devry Brasil (FANOR). Geoprocessing Analyst at the Fortaleza Municipal Health Department.

Isabelle Cordeiro de Nojosa Sombra
Nurse. Master in Collective Health (UECE). Specialist in Public Health (UECE). Lecturer at the Estácio do Ceará University Centre.

Jéssica Karen de Oliveira Maia
Nurse. Specialised in Nephrology Nursing (UECE).

José Auricélio Bernardo Cândido
Nurse. Master in Family Health (UECE). Specialist in Family Health (UFC). Specialist in Professional Health Education: Nursing (ENSP-FIOCRUZ). Specialist in Clinical Practices in Family Health (ESP-CE).

Juliana Alencar Moreira Borges
Nurse. Master in Public Health (UECE). Specialist in Health Services and Systems (FIOCRUZ). Specialist in Health Surveillance (UFC). Lecturer at the Estácio do Ceará University Centre.

Katherine Jeronimo Lima
Nurse. Master's student in Collective Health (UECE). Specialist Resident in Public Health (ESP/CE). Specialist in Health Care Network Management (FIOCRUZ). Specialist in Epidemiology (UFG).

Lídia Samara de Castro Sanders
Nurse. Master's in Collective Health (UECE). Specialist in Urgency and Emergency (ESP-CE), Stomatherapy Nursing (UECE) and Epidemiology and Health Surveillance (UFC). Lecturer on the Urgency and Emergency Training Course for SUS professionals (ESP/CE).

Lorena Samilla Sales Lucas
Nutritionist. Graduated from the Estácio do Ceará University Centre.

Mara Iza Holanda de Almeida
Nutritionist. Graduated from the Estácio do Ceará University Centre.

Maria Irismar de Almeida
Nurse. PhD in Nursing (UFC). Master's in Education (UFC). Nurse for the Ceará State Government and adjunct professor at the State University of Ceará.

Maria José Alves Anacleto
Nurse and Pedagogue. Specialist in Urgency and Emergency (FASP).

Maria Rosilene Cândido Moreira
Nurse. PhD in Biotechnology (RENORBIO/UFPB). Master's in Collective Health (UNIFESP). Specialist in Family Health, Collective Health and Nursing Education. Adjunct Professor at the Federal University of Cariri (UFCA). Permanent lecturer and Coordinator of the Postgraduate Programme in Sustainable Regional Development at UFCA (Proder).

Maura Vanessa Silva Sobreira
Nurse. PhD student in Health Sciences (FCMSC). Master's in Nursing (UFRN). Adjunct lecturer at the State University of Rio Grande do Norte (UERN).

Moacir Tavares Martins Filho
Dentist. PhD in Public Health from USP. Master in Public Health (UECE). Adjunct Professor at the Federal University of Ceará.

Priscila Nunes Costa Travassos
Nurse. Specialising in Nephrology Nursing (UECE) and Specialising in Intensive Care Nursing (UNIFOR).

Regina de Carvalho Kinjo
Medical doctor. Specialist in Neonatology at the Ceará School of Public Health (ESP-CE).

Rôsicler Pereira de Gois
Medical doctor. Master in Public Health (UECE). Resident in Neonatology (Albert Sabin Children's Hospital), Paediatrics (Fortaleza General Hospital) and General and Community Medicine (UFRN). Neonatologist at Albert Sabin Children's Hospital and on-call doctor at Antônio Prudente Hospital.

Radmila Alves Alencar Viana
Physiotherapist. Master's student in Collective Health (UECE). Resident specialising in Women's and Children's Health (UFC). Specialist in Public Health (UECE).

Selma Antunes Nunes Diniz
Nurse. Master's in Collective Health (UECE). Specialist in Auditing and Management of Health Systems and Hospitals (FIC). Specialist in Pedagogical Training in Professional Education (UFC).

Thamyres Fortaleza Monteiro
Nutrition student at the Estácio do Ceará University Centre.

Vinícius Ramalho Dantas Araújo
Resident Neonatologist at the Albert Sabin Children's Hospital.

Wenya Sarmento Sobrinho
Undergraduate student in Social Work at the Faculty of Philosophy, Sciences and Letters of Cajazeiras (FAFIC).

Weslley Epifanio Sarmento
Physiotherapist, Physical Educator and Pedagogue. Master's student in Agroindustrial Systems (UFCG). Specialist in Family Health (UFPB). Specialist in Health Management (UFRN).

SUMMARY

INTRODUCTION

Collective Health research in Brazil has achieved notable prominence. The approaches, methods and types of research are diverse and represent the relevance of this field: interdisciplinarity and transdisciplinarity.

In Ceará, scientific research models using a quantitative approach have been gaining ground for discussion within the Postgraduate Programme in Collective Health (PPSAC) at the State University of Ceará (UECE), through the Population Health Situation Research Line, one of the lines that guides studies in the Master's and Doctorate in Collective Health of the aforementioned Programme.

In this context, this book brings together contributions from authors, students and former students of the aforementioned Postgraduate Programme. Thus, the chapters that make up this book are the result of dissertations by PPSAC graduates, members and **former members of the Research Group "Evaluation and Statistical Analysis** in Public Health - **PESQSAÚDE", coordinated by professor and one of the** organisers of this book, Dr Francisco José Maia Pinto.

The book is organised into twelve chapters. Each chapter presents a different theme, but they are integrated by their research methodologies, analysis and epidemiological approach, given the various themes covered here.

Chapters 01, 02 and 03 deal with a serious public health problem in Brazil, the complications of drug use for maternal and neonatal health, and the discussion is based on quantitative approaches.

Chapter 04 discusses another important problem in the field of public health: congenital syphilis. The factors involved in morbidity and mortality due to vertical transmission of syphilis, and a description of the socio-economic, behavioural, gestational and treatment profiles of mothers and their partners are covered in these chapters, respectively.

Chapter 05 describes the characteristics of mothers and live births with congenital malformations in the municipality of Fortaleza-CE, in the period between
2001 a 2010. Chapter 06 analyses the epidemiological profile of infant mortality in the same municipality between 2005 and 2010.

Chapters 07 and 08 present an observational, cross-sectional and descriptive study carried out in a tertiary paediatric hospital in the state of Ceará, in order to address the profile of opioid use in a neonatal intensive care unit, and the criteria for the indication of packed red blood cells in a neonatal ICU, respectively.

Chapter 09 analyses the data from the Cervical Cancer Information System (SISCOLO) in the 16ª Health Region of Ceará - Camocim.

Chapters 10 and 11 deal with fundamental themes for promoting humanised care in Primary Health Care. These themes are the investigation of users' perceptions of reception and the identification of favourable and unfavourable conditions in the reception of users by the Family Health Strategy Team in Cajazeiras, Paraíba, Brazil; and the discussion of the importance of exclusive breastfeeding in the development of newborns, respectively.

Chapter 12 provides a relevant study of factors associated with the risk of developing type 2 diabetes mellitus.

As such, this book is made up of 12 chapters that discuss relevant issues in order to draw up an epidemiological profile of the state's main health problems. The perspectives of the researchers are multiple and, at the same time, converge to strengthen the field of Collective Health.

Happy reading!!!

Francisco Regis da Silva
Débora Sâmara Guimarães Dantas
Rafaella Maria Monteiro Sampaio
Francisco José Maia Pinto

CHAPTER 1

THE USE OF ILLICIT DRUGS DURING PREGNANCY AND OBSTETRIC COMPLICATIONS IN A MATERNITY HOSPITAL IN NORTH-EASTERN BRAZIL

Radmila Alves Alencar Viana

Francisco José Maia Pinto

Rafaella Maria Monteiro Sampaio

Katherine Jeronimo Lima

INTRODUCTION

Pregnancy is a physiological phenomenon that involves physical, social and emotional changes and should be seen as a healthy life experience. However, for some pregnant women, this experience can be marked by risk factors, which can increase the likelihood of an unfavourable outcome, thus generating a high-risk pregnancy (BRASIL, 2012).

Currently in Brazil, drug abuse and addiction have become major public health problems, aggravated by the association between motherhood and chemical substances. Even without official figures, the reality in hospitals draws attention to this problem; what was once an exception can now be seen as routine (OLÍVIO; GRACZVK, 2012).

A 2002 study found that 3% of American pregnant women aged between 15 and 44 had exposed their foetuses to one or more illicit drugs, with cocaine being the third most consumed drug by pregnant women, after marijuana and amphetamines (LUCCA, 2012).

Brazilian studies, such as the 6th National Survey on the Consumption of Psychotropic Drugs among Primary and Secondary School Students in Public and Private Schools, carried out in 2010, whose sample consisted of 50,890 students (CARLINI et al, 2010), revealed that between the genders, drug use is increasingly frequent among the female population. Drug use increases with age, which means that the age group considered fertile among women is compromised by the use of these substances.

Recently, between 2011 and 2013, another nationwide study of 7,381 drug users who reported using drugs on 25 days or more in the last 6 months revealed a growing number of female drug users in different age groups. The 18 to 24 and 35 to 39 age groups were the ones with the highest number of female crack and/or similar drug users compared to the male population (BASTOS; BERTONI, 2014).

This shows that the association between pregnancy and drug use is quite common in our society, whether in the younger age groups, as shown in the research among students, or in the older age groups, as shown in the research on crack cocaine. What we can conclude from analysing these two studies is that women and their fertile period are compromised when the use of licit and illicit substances is associated with pregnancy.

A retrospective study (MBAH et al, 2012) of 1,693,197 women identified various risks during pregnancy in cocaine users, including: placental abruption, oligoamnion, placental infarction, gestational hypertension, pre-eclampsia and eclampsia.

The main researcher's professional experience in a programme developed at a Maternity School prompted this research. The experience pointed to the need for research into this group of pregnant women, since they need comprehensive assistance and differentiated care, as well as initiatives that indicate ways of coping with drug use during pregnancy, in order to avoid and/or minimise maternal and neonatal complications.

This study aims to identify the use of illicit drugs among pregnant women and possible gynaecological/obstetric complications.

METHODS

This was a cross-sectional study with a quantitative-descriptive approach, carried out in a Maternity School located in the north-east of Brazil. The data was collected from the medical records of the puerperal women who gave birth between January and June 2015 at the maternity hospital and began after approval by the Ethics Committee with opinion number 1.215.261.

The population was made up of puerperal women who were illicit drug users admitted to the Maternity Hospital between January and June 2015, using secondary data from their medical records. The sample consisted of properly completed medical records with all the information relating to the study's objectives. Mothers who only used alcohol and/or tobacco during their current pregnancy were excluded from the study.

A structured form was used to collect data from the mothers' medical records. The form provided socioeconomic and demographic data on the mothers, obstetric and gynaecological history and data on the current pregnancy, such as the history of drug use during pregnancy and information on maternal complications and complications.

The variables relating to the proposed objectives were classified as outcome and explanatory. The outcome variable was represented by the use of illicit drugs during the current pregnancy in the group of puerperal women and the explanatory variables by the risk factors distributed in four hierarchical blocks, according to the conceptual model, which seeks to identify among the explanatory variables those that are most related to the outcome.

The explanatory variables were:

Block 1 - distal level: characteristics of the mother's socioeconomic and demographic profile

These are considered more distant from the model, since most of the time their effects are no longer statistically significant in the presence of intermediate and proximal level variables (LIMA; CARVALHO; VASCONCELOS, 2008).

- Marital status (single, married, civil partnership, divorced, widowed);
- Origin (capital, interior, other state);
- You work (yes, no);
- Schooling (no schooling, primary school, secondary school and higher education);
- Housing (own, not own, homeless);

Block 2 - intermediate level I: maternal characteristics, reproductive history, maternal morbidity and maternal behaviour:

These variables make up the intermediate level because they have effects whose magnitude is reduced when proximal variables are included (LIMA; CARVALHO; VASCONCELOS, 2008).

- Maternal age;
- Number of pregnancies (primigravida, multigravida);
- Previous abortion (yes, no);
- Previous obstetric complications (yes or no);

Block 3 - Intermediate II: characteristics relating to prenatal care and childbirth:

This level presents variables that have more significant effects on the outcome:

- Number of antenatal care visits (< 6, > 6);
- Type of birth (caesarean, vaginal, forceps);
- Positive tests on admission to labour (syphilis, HIV, toxoplasmosis, rubella, among others)

Block 4 - proximal: mother's health conditions and history of drug use during pregnancy:

The variables at the proximal level are the main ones responsible for the outcome.

- Type of drug used during pregnancy (crack, alcohol, cigarettes, cannabis, mixed, cocaine, other);
- Current obstetric complications (urinary tract infection, preterm labour, premature amniorrexia, HED, haemorrhages, others);

The SPSS programme version 17.0 was used to process the general data, while the EXCELL programme was used to store and construct graphs. The general data was analysed descriptively using frequencies (absolute and percentage). The inferential analysis was carried out with the variables hierarchised from the distal to the proximal model and grouped into two blocks. In each block, the association between the outcome and the explanatory variables was checked using the non-parametric chi-squared test at a significance level of 5%. The strength of the association between the variables was calculated using the odds ratio (OR), obtained by logistic regression analysis, which also adjusted for possible confounding effects.

RESULTS

The study's data collection consisted of 31 puerperal women who were illicit drug users. The puerperae were between 13 and 29 years old and were categorised into two groups, the first comprising adolescents and young adults and the other comprising only adults, according to the classification of the Brazilian Institute of Geography and Statistics (IBGE). As a result, the majority of puerperal women found were in the adolescent and young adult category, accounting for 54.8% (n = 17) compared to 45.2% (n = 14) of adults between 25 and 29 years of age (Table 1).

In terms of race/colour, all the puerperae in the study were classified **as "non-**

white", with 90.3% (n = 28) being brown and only 9.7% (n = 3) black. As for marital status, 58.1% (n = 18) were single and 41.9% (n = 13) were in a stable union. The majority of puerperal women came from the capital, representing 80.6% (n = 25) and 19.4% (n = 6) from the countryside (Table 1).

In terms of socio-economic profile, only 16.1% (n = 5) of the women had a paid job and the remaining 83.9% (n = 26) had no economic occupation. Low levels of education also prevailed in this group, with 93.5% (n = 29) of the puerperal women having primary education, which here includes both complete and incomplete primary education, and only 6.5% (n = 2) having secondary education, which also includes complete or incomplete secondary education (Table 1).

Table 1: Sociodemographic and socioeconomic profile of puerperal users. Fortaleza, 2015.

Sociodemographic profile			**Socio-economic profile**		
Age	N	%	**Does the pregnant woman work?**	N	%
13 a 24	17	54,8	Yes	5	16,1
25 a 29	14	45,2	No	26	83,9
Race			**Pregnant woman's schooling**		
Black	3	9,7	Elementary School	29	93,5
Brown	28	90,3	High School	2	6,5
Marital status			**Does the pregnant woman have a home?**		
Single	18	58,1	Own	9	29
Stable Union	13	41,9	Not Owned	22	71
Pregnant woman's origin					
Inside	6	19,4			
Capital	25	80,6			

Source: Author (2015)

Among the puerperal women who used illicit drugs who gave birth at the maternity school, 71% (n = 22) did not have their own home, three of whom lived on the streets and only 29% (n = 9) had their own home.

When the gynaecological and obstetric profile was investigated, it was found that 64.5% (n = 20) were multigravidas and among the 31 puerperal women who used illicit drugs, 35.5% (n = 11) had suffered abortions in a pregnancy prior to the study, 38.7% (n = 12) also had obstetric complications in previous pregnancies and the vast majority 74.2% (n = 23) suffered obstetric complications in the current pregnancy. With regard to the current pregnancy, 67.7% (n = 21) delivered vaginally (Table 2).

Table 2: Gynaecological and obstetric profile of puerperal users. Fortaleza, 2015.

Gynaecological and obstetric profile		
Number of pregnancies	N	%
Primigesta	11	35,5
Multigesta	20	64,5
Has there been a previous abortion?		
Yes	11	35,5
No	20	64,5
Current type of labour		
Caesarean section	10	32,3
Vaginal	21	67,7
Have there been any previous obstetric complications?		
Yes	12	38,7
No	19	61,3
Have there been any current obstetric complications?		
Yes	23	74,2
No	8	25,8
Did you carry out prenatal care?		
Yes	23	74,2
No	8	25,8
Number of prenatal consultations		
Less than 6 or None	23	74,2
More than 6	8	25,8
Positive tests		
Syphilis	16	51,6
None	15	48,4

Source: Author (2015)

Adherence to prenatal consultations was considered low in 74.2% (n = 23) of the puerperal women in the study, who had no or less than 6 prenatal consultations, and only 25.8% (n = 8) had more than 6 prenatal consultations. With regard to the tests carried out during admission for delivery and therefore recorded in the delivery report of the maternity hospital under study, 51.6% (n = 16) of these women tested positive for syphilis and 48.4% (n = 15) did not test positive for any of the other tests carried out at the time of delivery (Table 2).

The most common obstetric complications in the study were: urinary tract infection, haemorrhages, ruptured sacs, premature amniorrexia, oligoamnion, pre-eclampsia and malnutrition (Graph 1).

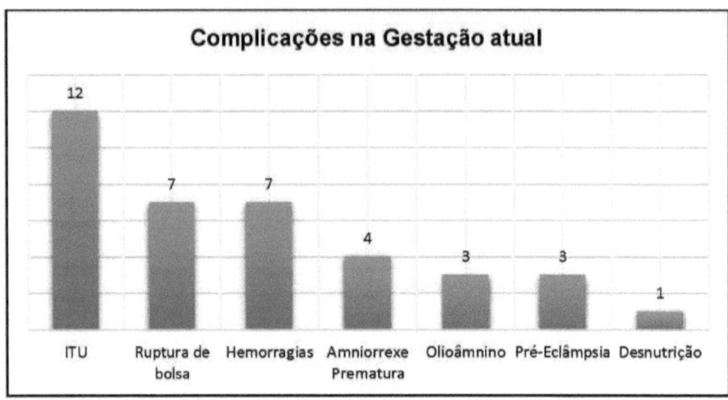

Graph 1: Complications in current pregnancy. Fortaleza, 2015.

Source: Author (2015)

When asked about the use of drugs during the current pregnancy, 80.6% (n = 25) of these women used three or more concomitant drugs during their pregnancy and 19.4% (n = 6) used up to two substances during pregnancy, at least one of which was considered an illicit drug.

When the test for variables was used to test the association between the use of illicit drugs during pregnancy and socioeconomic, demographic, gynaecological and obstetric profiles, no statistical significance was found ($p>0.05$).

DISCUSSION

According to the socio-demographic profile, the difference between the two age groups is minimal. What is worth highlighting, however, is the significant number of adolescents and young people using psychoactive substances in

our society. This data was not only found in the research presented here, but it is a reality that is very much present today.

It is known that adolescence is a stage of development that raises major concerns about drug use, as it is a time of exposure and vulnerability to drugs. It is a phase marked by biological, cognitive, emotional and social changes that are important for establishing and consolidating habits in adult life. It is generally during this period that experimentation with substances such as alcohol and other illicit drugs occurs

(PINHEIRO; PICANÇO; BARBEITO, 2011).

A nationwide survey found a large number of girls experimenting with illicit drugs at an early age. According to the survey, there was a higher prevalence at the age of 13 and 14, especially among girls, while boys stood out from the age of 15 or more. Girls consumed more in the last 30 days than boys, but without statistical significance (MALTA et al, 2011).

Thus, it can be said that the prevalent age group in this study corresponds to other studies. This demonstrates the need to strengthen public policies and intersectoral actions aimed at preventing drug use among young people, given the relevance of the problem.

The survey found a greater number of single women, which is in line with the results of other studies that also found a predominance of single, separated and widowed women among users (MELO et al, 2014). The national survey on crack also found that the majority (60.64 per cent) of crack and/or similar users in Brazil were single (BASTOS; BERTONI, 2014).

It can therefore be seen that single marital status in the case of female drug users can be considered an indicator of unstable family ties, which is often also a risk factor for the onset of drug use and its permanence throughout adulthood.

When asked about the employment situation of the puerperal women, 83.9% (n = 26) of them said they did not have any kind of income. This was similar to the findings of the study on the triggers of drug abuse in women, which found that none of the women interviewed **were in paid employment and that two of them were in a "street situation". In this same study,** low schooling, lack of employment, the presence of drugs in the community, the influence of friends, family and partners **were considered to be triggers for** the use of drugs of abuse (MARANGONI; OLIVEIRA, 2013).

Another study also stated that low income is seen as a contributing factor to the use of psychoactive substances, along with mental disorders, unemployment and a lack of stability in the civil partnership (THIENGO et al, 2012).

In this study, most of the women only had primary schooling, which means that low schooling in this group is a very common factor, and can also be seen as something that predisposes them to start using drugs.

Silva et al. (2014) found that the imbalance between schooling and age group may alert us to a possible cause or consequence relationship for the consumption of these substances, since low levels of schooling and difficulty in engaging in school have a strong potential to represent a vulnerability factor among adolescents and young adults, interfering with their integration and permanence in school and work.

Regarding the question of whether the pregnant woman had a home, 71% **(n=22) of them did not have their own home, as three of them were "homeless". It is understood that being in a "street situation" is another aggravating** factor **for the** condition of maternal and child life, since drug use is already a major detrimental factor, which combined with the fact that the pregnant woman/puerperal **woman is in a "street situation" makes the situation even worse, increasing** her vulnerability in various aspects, such as malnutrition, violence, among others that expose mother and newborn in a totally fragile context, which can have negative repercussions for the baby's future development.

Living on the streets is often due to weakened family ties. In a study on the lifestyles of the homeless population, it was found that a characteristic of almost all the groups is: low schooling, unemployment, no fixed address, migration from large metropolises and a strong relationship with drug use (KUNZ; HECKERT; CARVALHO, 2014).

With regard to the gynaecological and obstetric profile, the majority of puerperal women were multigravidae, which may represent an indicator of lack of family planning, since the situation of drug addiction associated with various conditions of social and economic vulnerability predispose them to unplanned pregnancies. This is often due to the occurrence of sexual violence, to which these women are exposed, or sex in exchange for drugs without adequate protection, which also makes them more susceptible to sexually transmitted diseases.

It is recognised that the choice to become pregnant is the result of the exercise of autonomy and reproductive freedom, so that an unplanned pregnancy is the result of a process in which the conscious decision of the woman or couple is absent. Socioeconomically unfavourable women who don't know their reproductive rights, contraception is a problem. Research shows that brown and black women with low levels of schooling and low family income, who have restricted access to contraceptives and little power to negotiate the use of condoms with their partners, are more exposed to unplanned pregnancies (COELHO et al, 2012).

As for the occurrence of miscarriage, 35.5 per cent (n=11) of these women had suffered a previous miscarriage, and this outcome may be related to drug use and therefore to complications in past pregnancies that culminated in miscarriage.

It is known that the use of drugs during pregnancy can cause changes in the uterus' ability to contract, in some cases leading to premature placental abruption (PPD), abnormal bleeding and even miscarriage (CAMARGO; MARTINS, 2014).

The most prevalent obstetric complications in this study were urinary tract infection, haemorrhage, ruptured sacs, premature amniorrexia, oligoamnion, pre-eclampsia and malnutrition.

A bibliographic study found that maternal complications from crack/cocaine use include premature labour, placental abruption, spontaneous abortion, cardiac dysrhythmias, liver rupture, cerebral ischaemia, heart attack and death, It is therefore estimated that preterm labour occurs in 17-29% of all pregnancies among crack and cocaine users, while in the general population it is 5-10% (HOLZTRATTNER, 2010).

Another issue that comes up a lot when studying drugs during pregnancy is the differential diagnosis, as patients who develop hypertension during pregnancy should be investigated for pre-eclampsia and acute intoxication, since both complications have similar symptoms and the use of beta-blockers in this group of patients is prohibited due to uncontrolled alpha adrenergic hyperstimulation following use of the medication, associated with worsening of the cardiovascular effects induced by cocaine (MARTISN-COSTA et al, 2013).

When the question was asked about prenatal care among the puerperal women, only 25.8% (n = 8) had more than six visits.

According to the Ministry of Health's prenatal care booklet, the main indicator of prognosis at birth may be access to prenatal care, and its early start is essential for adequate care, but the ideal number of visits remains controversial. According to the World Health Organisation (WHO), the appropriate number would be six (6) or more, but a reduced number of appointments (with greater emphasis on the content of each one) in cases of low-risk patients may not increase adverse perinatal outcomes. [a]Special attention should therefore be paid to pregnant women at higher risk (recommendation grade A), with monthly appointments up to the 28th week, fortnightly appointments between 28 and 36 weeks and weekly appointments at term (BRASIL, 2012a).

We can point out here that pregnant women who use illicit drugs are classified as high-risk pregnant women, as they are subject to numerous social, psychological and physiological aggravations.

According to the technical manual on high-risk pregnancy, the most common psychiatric conditions during pregnancy are mood disorders, anxiety disorders, psychotic disorders, abuse and dependence on psychoactive substances and eating disorders. There are therefore many negative consequences of illicit drug use, such as physical health problems, malnutrition and susceptibility to infections, which can be passed on to the developing foetus. However, the biggest problem in assessing the direct effects of illicit drugs on the foetus is the huge number of sociodemographic, psychosocial, behavioural and biological risk factors that are related to drugs and the consequences of unwanted pregnancy, such as poverty, lack of prenatal care, **STDs, malnutrition**, among others (BRASIL, 2012b).

When evaluating the positive tests, which were carried out at the time of admission for labour in the maternity hospital, 51.6% (n = 16) of the pregnant women tested positive for syphilis, a fact that was caused by a lack of quality prenatal care.

A study on the use of illicit drugs by HIV-infected pregnant women found that vertical transmission of the virus occurred more frequently in the newborns of pregnant women who used illicit drugs. According to the same study, drug use has been associated with an increase in the prevalence of unplanned pregnancies and sexually transmitted diseases (MELO et al, 2014).

This is probably due to the small size of the sample, as well as the fact that the notification service for pregnant drug users is not yet effective at the maternity hospital under study, and there is no data on this issue at the hospital. What we do have is data that is still being compiled by a study and action group that began in 2012 and has been consolidating itself. At the moment, this group is part of a recent strategy implemented at the hospital, which I took part in as a resident at the maternity hospital, helping to consolidate the data under construction.

CONCLUSION AND RECOMMENDATIONS

It can therefore be concluded that the results presented are similar to those of other studies looking at the profile of illicit substance users in the general population, while there are few national studies looking at drug use and pregnant women.

Despite the limited sample size, this study can contribute initial data on puerperal women treated at the maternity school and encourage other institutions to provide data on this population of women, who are often underreported, failing to offer more effective health policies and strategies for these pregnant drug users, which are increasingly growing in our society.

Efforts should therefore be made to ensure that other regions and localities carry out studies, notify and quantify these women, as well as drawing attention to strategies for welcoming, caring for and establishing links with this more socially fragile population, which therefore deserves a more specialised approach from the health team. In addition, the study of the consequences of intrauterine drug use on newborns should also be investigated in future studies, whether at primary care, outpatient or hospital level, so that health policies can reach this population.

National studies should be carried out on this population and their NBs, going beyond the data provided by institutional, regional or state studies in the literature. There is also a need for studies with larger samples so that statistically significant inferences and associations can be made.

All levels of health care should be alert to drug use during pregnancy, especially primary health care, which is considered the gateway and coordinator of health care networks, and should therefore carry out education and harm reduction actions so that pregnant drug users can have a pregnancy without complications.

REFERENCES

BASTOS, F.I.; BERTONI, N. (Org.). **National survey on crack use:** Who are the crack and/or similar users in Brazil? How many are there in the Brazilian capitals? Rio de Janeiro: Icict/fiocruz, 2014. 224 p.

BRAZIL. Ministry of Health. Low-risk prenatal care: Basic Care Notebooks, No. 32. Brasília: Editora do Ministério da Saúde, 2012a. 320 p. (Series A. Normas e Manuais Técnicos).

BRAZIL. Ministry of Health. High Risk Pregnancy: Technical Manual. 5. ed. Brasília: Editora Ms, 2012b. 302 p. (Series A - Standards and Technical Manuals).

CAMARGO, P.O.; MARTINS, M.F.D. The effects of crack on pregnancy and babies born to mothers who use it: A literature review. **Cadernos de Terapia Ocupacional**, Pelotas, v.1, n. 22, p.161-169, 2014.

CARLINI, E.L.A. et al (Org.). **VI National Survey on the Consumption of Psychotropic Drugs among Primary and Secondary School Students in the Public and Private Schools in the 27 Brazilian Capitals.** Brasília: Cebrid - Centro Brasileiro de Informações Sobre Drogas Psicotrópicas/ Unifesp - Universidade Federal de São Paulo/ Senad - Secretaria Nacional de Políticas Sobre Drogas, 2010. 503 p.

COELHO, E.A.C. et al. Association between unplanned pregnancy and the socioeconomic context of women in a Family Health Strategy area. **Acta Paulista de Enfermagem,** São Paulo, v.25, n.3, p.415-422, 2012.

HOLZTRATTNER, J.S. Crack cocaine, pregnancy, childbirth and the puerperium: a bibliographical study on care for users. 2010. 59 f. TCC (Graduation) - Nursing Course, Federal University of Rio Grande do Sul, Rio Grande do Sul, 2010.

KUNZ, G.S.; HECKERT, A.L.; CARVALHO, S.V. Modos de vida da população em situação de rua: inventando táticas nas ruas de Vitória/ES. Fractal, **Revista Psicologia**, Rio de Janeiro, v.26, n.3, p. 919-942, 2014.

LIMA, S.; CARVALHO, M.L.; VASCONCELOS, A.G.G. Proposal for a hierarchical model applied to the investigation of risk factors for neonatal infant death. **Cadernos de Saúde Pública**, Rio de Janeiro, v.24, p.1910-1916, 2008.

LUCCA, J. Ultrasound findings in the brains of newborns exposed to crack cocaine during pregnancy. 2012. 66 f. Master's Thesis - Master's Programme

in Medicine, Department of Paediatrics and Child Health, Pontifical Catholic University of Rio Grande do Sul, Porto Alegre, 2012.

MALTA, D.C.; et al. Prevalence of alcohol and drug consumption among adolescents: analysis of data from the National Health Survey
School. **Revista Brasileira de Epidemiologia**, Brasília, v.1, n.14, p.136-146, 2011.

MARTISN-COSTA, S.H.; et al. Crack: the new obstetric epidemic. **Revista Hcpa**, Porto Alegre, v.33, n.1, p.55-65, 2013.

MBAH A.K.; et al. Association between cocaine abuse in pregnancy and placenta associated syndromes using propensity score matching approach. **Early Hum Dev**, v.88, n.6, p.333-7, 2012.

MARANGONI, S.R.; OLIVEIRA, M.L.F. Factors triggering the use of drugs of abuse in women. **Texto e Contexto Enfermagem**, Florianópolis, v.3, n.22, p.662-70, 2013.

MELO, V.H.; et al. Use of illicit drugs by pregnant women infected with the
HIV. **Revista Brasileira de Ginecologia e Obstetrícia**, Belo Horizonte, v.12, n.36, p.555-561, 2014.

OLÍVIO, M.C.; GRACZVK, R.C. Women crack users and motherhood: brief considerations. Proceedings of the 2nd Gender and Public Policy Symposium: State University of Londrina, 18 and 19 August 2011.

PINHEIRO, A.; PICANÇO, P.; BARBEITO, J. A realidade do consumo de drogas nas populações escolares. **Revista Portuguesa de Clinica Geral,** Espírito Santos, v.27, p.348-355, 2011.

SILVA, C.C. et al. Initiation and consumption of psychoactive substances among adolescents and young adults at the Anti-Drug Psychosocial Care Centre/CAPS-AD. **Ciência & Saúde Coletiva**, Bahia, v.3, n.18, p.737-745, 2014.

THIENGO, D.L.; et al. Depression during pregnancy: a study on the association between risk factors and social support among pregnant women. **Cadernos de Saúde Coletiva**, Rio de Janeiro, v.20, n.4, p.416-426, 2012.

CHAPTER 2

APPLICATION OF THE HIERARCHICAL MODEL FOR COMPLICATIONS IN THE EARLY NEONATAL PERIOD RELATED TO MATERNAL DRUG ADDICTION

Isabelle Cordeiro de Nojosa Sombra

Francisco José Maia Pinto

Débora Sâmara Guimarães Dantas

Francisco Regis da Silva

Rafaella Maria Monteiro Sampaio

INTRODUCTION

The use of drugs, including alcohol, cigarettes, cannabis, cocaine and crack cocaine, is a major public health problem that has an alarming impact on society (YAMAGUCHI et al., 2008; SOUZA; SANTOS; OLIVEIRA, 2012). In the case of pregnant women, this problem receives greater emphasis, given that exposure to drugs can lead to irreversible impairment of the integrity of the mother and foetus, enabling the occurrence of miscarriage, premature birth, cognitive deficiencies in the conceptus and restricted foetal growth (AVERSI- FERREIRA et al., 2006; PASSINI, 2005; FREIRE; PADILHA; SAUNDERS, 2009). In addition, according to IBGE (2010), other physical health changes, malnutrition and susceptibility to infections can be passed on to the developing foetus.

The greatest difficulty in assessing the direct effects of drugs on the foetus is the large number of risk factors (sociodemographic, psychosocial, behavioural and biological) associated with poverty, lack of prenatal care, sexually transmitted diseases and malnutrition, which further compromises pregnancy, especially when it is unwanted (IBGE, 2010).

Drug use is one of the main risk factors involved in complications during pregnancy and childbirth. It can even be a determining cause of perinatal and neonatal mortality in newborns, and is a current problem of great public health relevance. Exposure to drugs by pregnant women has been a worldwide concern in terms of maternal and foetal health (BASTOS; BORNIA, 2009). Such exposure leads to perinatal complications, with emphasis on uteroplacental hypoperfusion, intrauterine growth retardation, premature placental abruption, increased incidence of premature rupture of membranes, as well as foetal malformations and miscarriages (YAMAGUCHI et al., 2008). The continuous and progressive use of these substances interrupts the physiological course of the body, leading to the development of pathologies, irreversible injuries and high rates of maternal mortality, stillbirth and neonatal mortality (LOPES; ARRUDA, 2010).

This study is an excerpt from Sombra's dissertation (2014) and aimed to analyse complications in the early neonatal period associated with maternal addiction to alcohol, cigarettes and other drugs in the municipality of Fortaleza-CE.

METHODS

This is a cross-sectional, descriptive and analytical study carried out in secondary care hospitals (Gonzaga Mota District Hospital in Messejana - HDGMM and Gonzaga Mota District Hospital in Barra do Ceará - HDGMBC) and tertiary care hospitals (Assis Chateaubriand Maternity School - MEAC, Fortaleza General Hospital - HGF and Dr César Cals General Hospital - HGCC) in the municipality of Fortaleza, which provide maternal and child health care, between March and May 2014.

The population consisted of all the mothers (5777) who were admitted to these hospitals with their respective children, corresponding to an average of 1909 births/month. The sample included all mothers **living in Fortaleza, with their respective NBs, who had been duly** hospitalised in the three months of the study and who had used at least one of the following drugs: licit (alcohol and cigarettes) and illicit (cannabis and cocaine/crack). Postpartum women with twin pregnancies and those with a diagnosed mental disorder (except drug addiction) were excluded. This exclusion was due to the possible confounding factor that could arise in relation to drug addiction, although this was treated as a type of mental disorder. The exclusion of twin pregnancies was due to the separation of the medical records of twin newborns, which were sometimes in different sectors, making data collection difficult.

To find the minimum sample size, the prevalence (10%) estimated through a pilot test, previously carried out, was considered, with a sampling error of 5%, at a significance level of 5%. The estimated sample size was 402 pregnant women/month. A further 29 pregnant women were added to compensate for possible sample losses, which amounted to just under 10%. Thus, the final sample consisted of 431 mothers, distributed in the five reference hospitals surveyed.

Data was collected after the birth of the child, using interviews with pregnant women. Two semi-structured forms were used, the first with the mothers and the second to collect information related to labour and birth from the mother's medical records.

In this study, the risk factors for complications in the early neonatal period were described and categorised using the hierarchical model, according to the adaptation of the conceptual model (LIMA; CARVALHO; VASCONCELOS, 2008).

The variables were analysed, with the outcome being the dichotomous variable referring to the occurrence of complications in the early neonatal period (yes, no).

Complications occurring in the early neonatal period included the variables neonatal dystocia, accidents and complications per se: acrocyanosis, cyanosis, respiratory distress, risk of meconium bronchoaspiration (BAM), risk of neonatal infection (INN), congenital cytomegalovirosis, neonatal jaundice, congenital malformation, risk of hypoglycaemia, macrosomia, risk of retrovirus, acute pneumopathy, risk of abstinence syndrome, upper limb ecchymosis, risk of toxoplasmosis, cardiomegaly, hypoactivity and risk of pulmonary hypertension, Down's syndrome, archaic reflexes, risk of maternal-fetal incompatibility (MFI-ABO), risk of congenital syphilis, congenital syphilis, heart murmur, absent gait reflex and foetal death (CUNHA et al., 2001).

The following variables were considered explanatory: the mother's socio-economic and socio-demographic characteristics; maternal characteristics including age, reproductive history, previous maternal morbidity and maternal behaviour; prenatal and childbirth care; NB health conditions and neonatal care provided, seen in four hierarchical blocks.

Initially, univariate data analysis was carried out to select the variables in each block, considering the descriptive level $p<0.20$. To identify the existence of an association between the outcome and the explanatory variables, the non-parametric Chi-squared test was used at a significance level of 5%. The strength of the association between the variables was measured by the odds ratio (OR, simple and adjusted), obtained from the logistic regression, which also adjusted for possible confounding effects. In the logistic regression, a descriptive level of $p<0.20$ was considered for the variable to be included in the regression model and a value of $p<0.05$ for this variable to remain in the model.

In the multivariate analysis, only the significant variables ($p<0.05$) were included, following the hierarchical models, according to the conceptual model (MOSLEY; CHEN, 1984). In this process, the variables in the distal blocks were introduced and, concomitantly, only the variables in the same block, followed by those included in the intermediate block, until reaching those in the proximal block (VICTORA et al., 1997). The hierarchisation technique not only makes precedence over time explicit, but also highlights the importance of different factors in the outcome, which exceeds the estimates of the traditional multiple regression statistical model (VASCONCELOS; ALMEIDA; NOBRE, 2001).

The study followed the recommendations of Resolution 466/12, which regulates research involving human beings. After receiving a favourable opinion, data collection began. The hospitals joined by presenting the approval report, 670.082 dated 21/03/2014, provided by CEP/UECE, to the head of the Research Centre.

The mothers signed the Free and Informed Consent Form (FICF), which informed them of their right not to take part or to withdraw from the study at any time. In the case of underage mothers, the ICF was signed by their guardian.

RESULTS

When we analysed the epidemiological profile of the study sample in relation to socioeconomic and demographic characteristics, we found that more than half of the mothers had secondary or higher education 254 (58.9%), an unpaid occupation 300 (69.6%) and, of those who had a paid occupation 131 (30.4%), only part had a formal employment contract 71 (16.5%). More than half of the mothers did not receive any government aid 298 (69.1%), had a family income of less than or equal to one minimum wage 332 (77%) and 282 (65.4%) were in a stable union.

With regard to maternal characteristics, reproductive history, previous maternal morbidity and maternal behaviour, it was observed that, according to the age of the participants in the sample, the majority of mothers (50.6%) were in the intermediate age group, from 20 to 29 years old (Md: 24.57; Dp: 6.779). In addition, the majority had no previous morbidity (93.5%), had positive **"O" blood** type (58%) and positive Rh factor (94.7%).

Analysing the number of pregnancies (Md: 2.32; SD: 1.809), we found that most of the sample was made up of multigravida mothers (54.3%), in contrast to the parity variable (Md: 2.03; SD: 1.489), which shows primiparous mothers in higher numbers (51%). This data was contradicted by the presence of miscarriages in previous pregnancies (Md: 0.28; SD: 0.565), suffered by 23.2 per cent of the mothers.

Serological tests for syphilis (VDRL) were mostly negative (70.8%), but it is worth noting that 64 puerperal women (14.8%) had still not been tested, even after giving birth. The serological test to identify HIV showed that the majority of mothers were seronegative (85.8), however, a small percentage had not undergone the test either (8.8%).

Among the mothers in the sample studied, some had used some kind of drug (licit or illicit) during pregnancy (13.4%). Among the drugs identified, tobacco was the most consumed (8.4%), followed by alcohol (7.4%) and illicit drugs (6.3%).

When we analysed the data relating to the characteristics of prenatal care, we found that the majority of mothers had prenatal care (93.5%) and started follow-up in the first trimester of pregnancy (62.6%); however, only some (55%) had 6 or more visits (Md: 5.68; SD: 2.686). Most of the mothers had received their prenatal care at the Basic Health Unit (UBS) (66.4%). With regard to childbirth, there was no spontaneous rupture of the sac in the majority of cases (61.7%) and the most common type of delivery was caesarean section (55.5%).

With regard to the health conditions of the newborn, it was observed that the **majority of NBs were** male (59.9%), born at term (81.2%) (Md: 38s5d; SD: 15.197), with an Adequate Gestational Age (AIG), (73.5%), in good condition at birth (66.1%), within the appropriate weight range (74.9%) (Md: 3013.6; SD: 656.868), with a height range of less than 50 cm (63.3%) (Md: 48.6%; SD: 2.874), with a WC range between 33 and 36 cm (67.3%): 656.868), height range less than 50 cm (63.3%) (Md: 48.21; SD: 2.874), WC range between 33 and 36cm (67.3%) (Md: 34.18; SD: 1.936), PT range less than 2cm in relation to WC (61.7%) (Md: 32.57; SD: 2.702), Apgar score in the first minute greater than or equal to 7 (89.6%) (Md: 8; SD: 1.372) and in the fifth minute also greater than or equal to 7 (99.5) (Md: 9; SD: 0.814). The **blood** type of **the majority of NBs was "O" (57.3%) and Rh positive (97.7%).**

When we analysed neonatal care, we found that **rehabilitation manoeuvres** were used on the **majority of NBs (82.6%) and most were** sent to rooming-in (87.9%).

Out of a total of 362 complications identified in this period, Early Respiratory Distress (ERD) stands out (29.3 per cent), followed by Risk of Neonatal Infection (RNI) (13 per cent) and Cyanosis (11.6 per cent).

Table 1: Adjusted distal risk factors for the development of complications in the early neonatal period, according to the socioeconomic and demographic characteristics of the mothers, Fortaleza, CE, BR, 2014.

VARIABLE	SAMPLE n(=431)	SAMPLE %	Gross OR	95% CI	P
Marital status					
Living in a stable union	282	65,4	1,0	1,06;2,39	0,025
Not in a stable union	149	34,6	1,59		

95% CI: 95% confidence interval; OR: Odds Ratio.
Source: Research data

Table 2: Intermediate risk factors I, adjusted for the development of complications in the early neonatal period, according to maternal characteristics, reproductive history, previous maternal morbidity and maternal behaviour, Fortaleza, CE, BR, 2014.

VARIABLES	SAMPLE n (=431)	SAMPLE %	OR gross	95% CI	P
Number of pregnancies					
Multigesta	234	54,3	1,0	0,92;1,99	0.116
Primigesta	197	45,7	1,35		
Licit and/or illicit drugs					
No	374	86.8	1,0	0,15;0,58	<0,001
Yes	57	13,2	0,30		
Smoking					
No	395	91,6	1,0	0,15;0,76	0,007
Yes	36	8,4	0,34		
Alcoholism					
No	399	92,6	1,0	0,14;0,79	0,010
Yes	32	7,4	0,33		
Illicit drugs					
No	405	94	1,0	0,006;0,34	<0,001
Yes	26	6	0,04		
VDRL					
Negative or not realised	369	85,6	1,0	1,53;5,49	0,001
Positive	62	14,4	2,90		
HIV					
Negative or not realised	408	94,5	1,0	1,08;5,90	0,040
Positive	23	5,5	2,46		

95% CI: 95% confidence interval; OR: Odds Ratio.
Source: Research data

Table 3: Intermediate risk factors II, adjusted for the development of complications in the early neonatal period, according to characteristics related to prenatal care and childbirth, Fortaleza, CE, BR, 2014.

SAMPLE

VARIABLES	n(=431)	%	Gross OR	95% CI	P
Did your antenatal care					
Yes	403	93,5	1,0	2,61;47,57	<0,001
No	28	6,5	11,14		
Number of antenatal appointments					
>6	237	55	1,0	1,45;3,29	<0,001
< 6	166	38,5	2.18		
Type of labour					
Normal	192	44,5	1,0	1,13;2,44	0,010
Caesarean section	239	55,5	1,66		

95% CI: 95% confidence interval; OR: Odds Ratio.
Source: Research data

Table 4: Proximal risk factors, adjusted for the development of complications in the early neonatal period, according to the newborn's health conditions and neonatal care, Fortaleza, CE, BR, 2014.

VARIABLES	SAMPLE		Gross OR	95% CI	P
	n(=431)	%			
Gestational age (weeks)					
RNT (from 37 to 41 weeks and 6 days)	350	81,2	1,0	0,19;0,59	<0,001
PTNB (< 37 weeks) or RNPOT (> 42 weeks)	80	18,8	0,33		
Gestational Age Classification					
AIG	317	73,5	1,0	0,29;0,73	0,001
PIG or GIG	114	26,5	0,46		
Conditions at birth					
Good	285	66,1	1,0	0,03;0,12	<0,001
Cyanosis and/or meconium	146	33,9	0,06		
Birth weight (grams)					
From 2501g to 4000g	323	74,9	1,0	1,32;3,68	0,002
< 2500g or > 4001g	106	25,1	2,21		
Apgar at the 1st minute					
Greater than or equal to 7	386	89,6	1,0	0,02;0,27	<0,001
Less than 7	45	10,4	0,08		

95% CI: 95% confidence interval; OR: Odds Ratio.
Source: Research data

Table 5: Predictive models for the development of early neonatal complications for four levels of hierarchy, Fortaleza, CE, BR, 2014

VARIABLES	Adjusted OR	95% CI	P
MODEL 1			
Distal block			

Marital status (non-stable union)	1,59	1,05;2,41	0,026
MODEL 2			
Distal block			
Marital status (non-stable union)	2,60	1,56;4,34	<0,001
Intermediate block I			
Illicit drugs (yes)	13,38	1,69;105,60	0,014
HIV (positive)	0,17	0,06;0,49	0,001
MODEL 3			
Distal block			
Marital status (non-stable union)	1,95	1,20;3,17	0,007
Intermediate block I			
Illicit drugs (yes)	7,08	0,81;61,37	0,075
HIV (positive)	0,19	0,07;0,56	0,002
Intermediate block II			
No. of prenatal consultations (< 6 enquiries)	2,67	1,67;4,28	<0,001
Type of delivery (caesarean)	2,94	1,83;4,74	<0,001
MODEL 4 (FINAL)			
Distal block			
Marital status (non-stable union)	1,93	1,11;3,34	**0,019**
Intermediate block I			
Illicit drugs (yes)	4,75	0,45;49,87	**0,193**
HIV (positive)	0,15	0,04;0,56	**0,004**
Intermediate block II			
No. of antenatal care visits (< 6 visits)	2,33	1,35;4,02	**0,002**
Type of delivery (caesarean)	3,03	1,78;5,13	**<0,001**
Proximal block			
Conditions at birth (Cyanosis and/or meconium)	9,71	4,93;19,13	**<0,001**
Gestational age classification (PIG or GIG)	0,37	0,20;0,66	**0,001**

95% CI: 95% confidence interval; OR: Odds Ratio.
Source: Research data

The model was confirmed by the Hosmer-Lemeshow statistic, which showed no significant difference between the predicted and observed variables, making it a good model.

DISCUSSION

In the distal block, it was observed that the mothers' marital status influenced the outcome. Most of the mothers were living with their partner, which was also important as a protective factor in relation to the development of early neonatal complications. A study of 408 adolescents in a municipality in São Paulo found different results, with 61 per cent of pregnant women not living with their boyfriend or husband (CAPUTO; BORDIN, 2008).

In intermediate block I, there was a significant association between illicit drug use and the outcome. The literature shows that exposure to drugs during pregnancy is a risk factor for newborn health, including neonatal death, mainly due to its teratogenic characteristics; however, some studies have found no statistical association between drug use and complications for newborn health (NASCIMENTO et al., 2012).

Drug use during pregnancy is a risk factor that can be avoided or minimised through prenatal care. This shows the importance of prenatal care, understanding that good monitoring favours a safer pregnancy, thereby avoiding maternal and foetal risks.

The medical records of most of the institutions studied did not contain information on the use of drugs other than alcohol and cigarettes in the standardised instrument. It was only possible to collect this information by interviewing the mothers and confirming it with loose information in the mother's/NB's medical records. It was felt that this aspect should be changed in order to enable more detailed studies on this very relevant issue, as there is an increasing number of drug users during the childbearing period who simply deny their use, thus making research on the subject more difficult, especially during data collection, which jeopardises obtaining reliable information.

Pregnant women may report less consumption or deny it in order to avoid possible reprimand and disapproval from health professionals. Health professionals must be sensitised to this reality, avoiding embarrassing women and gaining their trust in the search for reliable information (SOUZA; SANTOS; OLIVEIRA, 2012).

Also, in intermediate block I, the variable referring to seropositivity was significant in relation to the development of complications in the early neonatal period.

HIV infection has been associated with the use of illicit drugs during pregnancy (HEIL **et *al*.**, 2011). A study of 845 HIV-positive patients, when asked during prenatal consultations, only 64 (7.6%) said they had used illicit drugs at some point during pregnancy (MELO **et *al*.**, 2014). With regard to neonatal complications, cases of respiratory distress, sepsis, early jaundice and metabolic disorders were observed, **occurring more frequently among the NBs of pregnant users.**

The results of this study indicate improved access to prenatal care, which corroborates the findings of other studies (BASSO; NEVES; SILVEIRA, 2012). However, although adherence to follow-up has increased, it should also be taken into account whether the minimum number of appointments has been made, as it was observed that pregnant women who had fewer than six antenatal appointments had a higher risk of developing the outcome compared to those who had six or more appointments.

In Intermediate Block II, in relation to adherence to prenatal care by mothers, it was found that although more than half of the mothers attended prenatal care, there was low adherence in relation to the number of visits, with an average of only 3.69 visits throughout pregnancy, which is well below the WHO recommendation, as the number of visits is a good indicator of risk prevention. Starting prenatal care early and having at least six appointments contribute to the quality of follow-up. If fewer than seven visits are made, there is a 1.4 times greater chance of neonatal death. Similar results were found in a study outlining infant mortality in the state of São Paulo, which reported a significant reduction in the likelihood of death as the number of visits increased (ORTIZ; OUSHIRO, 2008).

Antenatal care is undoubtedly an essential factor in women's health care during pregnancy. By carrying out the recommended tests and monitoring foetal growth, it is possible to detect alterations that could cause maternal and foetal problems. During pregnancy, many changes occur in a woman's body, which means that this period requires special care. These are months of preparation for the birth of the child, and it is important that mothers-to-be are closely monitored in accordance with the prenatal care guidelines (SANTOS et al., 2009).

In intermediate block II, caesarean section was significantly associated with the risk factor for developing neonatal complications. Among the many guidelines given to women during prenatal care, the literature points to vaginal delivery as the one with the lowest risk to mother and foetus, and it should be indicated as the first option, because, except in cases where caesarean section is really necessary, vaginal delivery is considered the natural way to be born, and its complications are less serious than those resulting from surgical delivery. It is also with normal labour that breastfeeding becomes easier and healthier for the newborn, and hospital-acquired infections are much less frequent (QUEIROZ et al., 2005).

However, caesarean section, as the most frequent type of delivery, can be justified by the high incidence of hypertensive disorders during pregnancy, which are indicative of this type of procedure in order to preserve the lives of mother and baby. When properly indicated, caesarean section reduces anoxia and obstetric trauma, enabling a marked reduction in foetal and maternal mortality. The indication for caesarean section is valuable when it is carried out with the aim of saving lives and preventing sequelae (SANTOS et al., 2009).

In the proximal block, the variables relating to gestational age (GA) classification and birth conditions were statistically significant in relation to the outcome. A GA classified as PIG or GIG was associated with the occurrence of the outcome, as were children who presented cyanosis and/or were bathed in meconium shortly after birth.

In women with high-risk pregnancies, the incidence of meconium in the amniotic fluid (MLA) is between 10% and 16% in term deliveries. Meconium aspiration syndrome (MAS) is the main complication of MLA and a major cause of perinatal mortality. The mechanical and chemical effects and inflammatory responses caused by MAS can interfere with the normal transition to extrauterine life, causing airway obstruction, damage to lung tissue, surfactant inactivation, chemical pneumonitis and a decrease in arterial oxygen pressure. The most common causes of ALM include gastrointestinal maturity of the foetus, foetal response to hypoxia and intrauterine infection (OSAVA et al., 2012).

CONCLUSION

This issue is relevant because it is from this that the real situation of the problem can be assessed and a plan or strategy drawn up to intervene with a focus on caring for pregnant women. It was found that the majority of pregnant drug users were of reproductive age, which can be considered an aggravating factor.

In addition, there is little research on the use of licit and illicit substances by pregnant women, and it is difficult to carry out research focussing on drugs other than alcohol and cigarettes, as the approach to these mothers must be different. This can be seen in the fact that there are few sources of information, such as medical records, which do not contain this relevant information. This shows how much progress still needs to be made on this issue, both in terms of prevention, treatment and analysing the physical and social effects of drug use by pregnant women and its consequences for their newborns.

Prenatal care can be a great ally in reversing or alleviating this problem, since professionals can provide pregnant women with the necessary and sufficient information through prenatal care, since there is low adherence in this sector by pregnant users. To this end, it is necessary to train professionals in humanising care for women in this process, as well as being sensitive to perceiving risk, which can be essential to avoid future complications and neonatal deaths.

Some recommendations should be emphasised, including a focus on effective public health policy actions, such as: expanding the women's health care network, improving access to prenatal care for pregnant women and the quality of care; carrying out the tests recommended by the Ministry of Health and guaranteeing a referral maternity hospital for childbirth, thus avoiding women's pilgrimage. It is essential to seek improvements in order to avoid early neonatal complications, such as the use of licit and illicit drugs during pregnancy.

REFERENCES

AVERSI-FERREIRA TA; RODRIGUES HG; NERES AC; FONSECA LC; PENHA- SILVA N. Immunohistochemical study of the olfactory bulb of wistar rats submitted to acute prenatal exposure to ethanol. **Biosci J**., v.22; n.1, p.99-105, 2006.

BASSO CG; NEVES ET; SILVEIRA A. Association between prenatal care and neonatal morbidity. **Texto contexto Enfermagem**, v.21, n.2, p.269-276, 2012.

BASTOS MS; BORNIA ECS. **Use of nicotine and/or cocaine during pregnancy and its consequences for foetal and neonatal development.** V EPCC Encontro Internacional de Produção Científica Cesumar, 27 to 30 October 2009.

CAPUTO VG; BORDIN IA. Teenage pregnancy and frequent use of alcohol and drugs in the family context. **Revista de Saúde Pública**, v.42, n.3, p.402- 410, 2008.

CUNHA GB; et al . Prevalence of prenatal exposure to cocaine in a sample of newborns from a general university hospital. **Jornal de Pediatria**, v.77, n.5, p.369-373, 2001.

FREIRE K; PADILHA PC; SAUNDERS Cláudia. Factors associated with the use of alcohol and cigarettes during pregnancy. **Revista Brasileira de Ginecologia e Obstetrícia**, v.31, n.7, p.335-341, 2009.

HEIL SH; JONES HE; ARRIA A; KALTENBACH K; COYLE M; FISCHER G; et *al.* Unintended pregnancy in opioid-abusing women. **J Subst Abuse Treat,** v.40, n.2, p.199-202, 2011.

IBGE. **Brazilian Institute of Geography and Statistics**, 2010.

LIMA S; CARVALHO ML; VASCONCELOS AGG. Proposal for a hierarchical model applied to the investigation of risk factors for neonatal infant death. **Cadernos de Saúde Pública**, v.24, n.8, p.1910-1916, 2008.

LOPES TD; ARRUDA PP. The repercussions of drug abuse in the pregnancy/puerperal period. **Revista Saúde e Pesquisa**, v.3; n.1; p.79-83, 2010.

MELO VH; et *al.* Use of illicit drugs by HIV-infected pregnant women. **Revista Brasileira de Ginecologia e Obstetrícia**, v.36, n.12, p.555-561,2014.

MOSLEY WH; CHEN IC. Analytical framework for the study of child survival in developing countries. **Popul Dev Rev,** v.10, sl, p.25-45, 1984.

NASCIMENTO RM; et al. Determinants of neonatal mortality: a case-control study in Fortaleza, Ceará, Brazil. **Cadernos de Saúde Pública**, v.28, n.3, p.559-572, 2012.

ORTIZ LP; OUSHIRO DAkiko. Profile of Neonatal Mortality in the State of São Paulo. **São Paulo em Perspectiva**, v.22, n.1, p.19-29, 2008.

OSAVA RH; et al. Maternal and neonatal factors associated with meconium in amniotic fluid in a normal birth centre. **Revista de Saúde Pública**, v.46, n.6, p.1023-1029, 2012.

PASSINI JUNIOR R. Alcohol consumption during pregnancy. **Revista Brasileira de Ginecologia e Obstetrícia**, v.27, n.7, p.373-375, 2005.

QUEIROZ MVO; et al . Incidence and characteristics of caesarean sections and normal deliveries: a study in a city in the interior of Ceará. **Revista Brasileira de Enfermagem**, v.58, n.6, p.687-691, 2005.

SANTOS ZMSA; et al. Risk factors for pregnancy-specific hypertensive syndrome. **Revista Brasileira em Promoção da Saúde**, v.22, n.1, p.48-54, 2009.

SOMBRA ICN. **Maternal drug addiction and complications in the early neonatal period**: a hierarchical model. 2014. 92f. Dissertation (Master's in Collective Health) - State University of Ceará, Fortaleza, 2014.

SOUZA LHRF; SANTOS MC; OLIVEIRA LCM. Pattern of alcohol consumption among pregnant women treated at a public university hospital and associated risk factors. **Revista Brasileira de Ginecologia e Obstetrícia**, v.34, n.7, p.296- 303, 2012.

VASCONCELOS AGG; ALMEIDA RMV; NOBRE FF. Path analysis and multi-criteria decision making: an approach for multivariate model selection and analysis in health. **Ann Epidemiol,** v.11, p.377-84, 2001.

VICTORA CG; HULTTLY SR; FUCHS SC; OLINTO MTA. The role of conceptual frameworks in epidemiological analysis: a hierarchical approach. **Int J Epidemiol,** v.26, p.224-7, 1996.

YAMAGUCHI ET; et al. Drugs of abuse and pregnancy. **Revista de Psiquiatria Clínica**, v.35, supl.1, p.44-47, 2008.

CHAPTER 3

GESTATIONAL DRUG ADDICTION AND NEONATAL DEATH IN A BRAZILIAN CAPITAL: socieconomic, demographic and maternal characteristics under study

Juliana Alencar Moreira Borges
Selma Antunes Nunes Diniz
Geziel dos Santos de Sousa
Francisco José Maia Pinto
Francisco Regis da Silva
Débora Sâmara Guimarães Dantas
Rafaella Maria Monteiro Sampaio

INTRODUCTION

Among the various factors related to infant mortality, drug use during pregnancy stands out as a new factor, increasingly present in prenatal reports, and may even be associated with prematurity, low birth weight, reduced head circumference, placental abruption and other conditions related to death (PINHEIRO; LAPREGA; FURTADO, 2005).

Infant mortality covers deaths of children under 1 year old, and is divided into neonatal mortality - deaths from 0 to 27 days of life, and post-neonatal mortality - deaths from 28 days to 364 days of life. Neonatal mortality is subdivided into two periods, early neonatal mortality - 0 to 6 days of life, and late neonatal mortality - 7 to 27 days of life (BRASIL, 2009; GAIVA; BITTENCOURT; FUJIMORI, 2013a).

Brasil (2011) points out that neonatal mortality accounts for around 60 to 70 per cent of infant mortality and, therefore, greater advances in the health of Brazilian children require greater attention to the health of neonates.

In this sense, epidemiological studies show that infant mortality is higher in the neonatal component, hence the importance of improving prenatal care, childbirth care and the first days of the child's life. Studying the factors involved in neonatal deaths makes it possible to identify the profile, as well as the various variables related to the outcome (DANTAS, et al., 2014).

Among the variables that may be involved in neonatal death, such as birth weight, gestational age and family income, we highlight the use of drugs during pregnancy, now observed by health professionals as something growing among pregnant women and which can trigger premature births and neonatal deaths (GAIVA; FUJIMORI; SATO, 2014b).

Drug use and addiction is something that has existed for a long time and is not exclusive to modern society. According to Carranza and Pedrão (2005), it is an ancient and universal practice, and is therefore not a phenomenon exclusive to the times in which we live. It can therefore be said that the history of drug addiction is intertwined with the history of humanity itself.

Worldwide, around 200 million people - almost 5 per cent of the population aged between 15 and 64 - use illicit drugs at least once a year. The most widely consumed drug in the world is cannabis (marijuana and hashish) (UNODC, 2010).

In 2001, the First Household Survey on the Use of Psychotropic Drugs in Brazil was carried out, a study involving the 107 largest cities in the country, with the aim of drawing up a profile of drug use in Brazil (CARLINI et al., 2002).

In the second survey, in 2005, in Brazil, the use of any drug in life (except tobacco and alcohol) was 22.8 per cent. This percentage is, for example, close to Chile (23.4 per cent) and almost half that of the USA (45.8 per cent). The prevalence of using any drug in life, except tobacco and alcohol, was highest in the Northeast region, where 27.6 per cent of those interviewed had used some drug (CARLINI, 2006).

Thinking about the use of drugs by women, especially pregnant women, reveals yet another major challenge for public health, because in addition to the problems arising from this practice in the family context and women's health, the health and lives of children who may be born to drug-using mothers also come into play (GAIVA; FUJIMORI; SATO, 2014b).

Thus, according to Dantas et al. (2014), women play a fundamental role in society, due to the possibility of generating a child in their womb, allowing the continuity of the species. This process, which begins with fertilisation, lasts until the child becomes an adult, responsible for their actions. Therefore, drug use by pregnant women will have serious and sometimes irreversible consequences not only for the mother, but also for her offspring.

Based on discussions with the literature and the experiences of death surveillance and the Committee for the Prevention of Infant and Foetal Deaths of the Regional Executive Secretariat II, it was possible to observe that drug use during pregnancy is now present in several infant death investigations, confirming the increase in this practice by women during pregnancy.

Therefore, based on the above considerations, and considering that this study is an excerpt from the dissertation by Borges (2012), the aim was to outline the socioeconomic and demographic profile, as well as maternal characteristics, reproductive history, maternal morbidity and behaviour of the mothers under study, in Fortaleza, Ceará, between 2009 and 2010.

METHODS

This is a case-control study. Thus, the analytical method used, case-control, was chosen due to its importance in comparing two groups based on the frequency of exposure to the risk factor(s) of interest (RÊGO, 2010).

Through the two groups chosen, cases (neonatal deaths) and controls (live births surviving the neonatal period), the risk factors for the occurrence of neonatal death can be observed.

The study was carried out at the Assis Chateaubriand Maternity School - MEAC, in the municipality of Fortaleza, Ceará, with neonatal deaths and births that occurred in Fortaleza residents, from 1st January 2009 to 31st December 2010.

The study universe consisted of 9,450 children born alive at MEAC in 2009 and 2010. The population was made up of 7,389 (78.2%) mothers living in Fortaleza. During the same period, there were 251 neonatal deaths, of which 153 (61%) were Fortaleza residents (SMS - TABNET, Fortaleza).

The sample was made up of all 153 neonatal deaths (cases), and the controls (464) consisted of survivors of the neonatal period who were discharged from hospital and selected at random. The choice of three controls for each case was determined in order to increase the level of statistical certainty proposed by Mendes, Olinto and Costa (2006), who suggest that the proportion of just two controls for each case is sufficient to guarantee statistical power and, at the same time, not compromise efficiency.

The first data was collected using the linkage technique between the databases of deaths and births at MEAC, which are fed into the Mortality Information System (SIM) and the National Births System (SINASC). Data collection from hospital records began when the MEAC Ethics Committee issued its favourable opinion.

The variables covered were divided into blocks. Block 1 included characteristics of the mother's socio-economic and demographic profile: years of **schooling (<4 and >4 years of age); marital status (cohabiting,** not cohabiting); work (yes and no).

Block 2 included maternal characteristics, reproductive history, maternal **morbidity and maternal behaviour: maternal age (<20, > 20 years); gestational age (<37, > 37 weeks); type of pregnancy (single,** multiple); number of pregnancies (primigravida, multigravida); number of births (primipara, multipara); **number of abortions (none, 1, >2); (UTI) urinary tract infection (yes and no);** (SAH) systemic arterial hypertension (yes and no); drug use (yes and no); smoking during pregnancy (yes and no); alcohol during pregnancy (yes and no); and other drugs (yes and no).

The data was stored in the Microsoft Office Excel programme®, 2010, and processed using the STATA statistical programme, version 10.

Initially, a descriptive frequency analysis (absolute and relative values) and parametric analysis (mean and standard deviation) were carried out.

In each block, the association between the outcome (neonatal death) and the explanatory variables was checked using the non-parametric chi-square test at a 5% significance level.

The strength of the association between the variables was made possible by calculating the odds ratio (OR), obtained through logistic regression analysis, which also adjusted for possible confounding effects. Possible confounding effects were then controlled by oscillating the OR up or down by 10 per cent.

The use of logistic regression considered the descriptive level $p<0.20$ for inclusion in the regression model and the value of $p<0.05$ for the variable to remain in the model. Finally, multiple regression was carried out only with the significant variables ($p<0.05$) of each hierarchical block in the study of neonatal mortality (VICTORA et al., 1997).

The final analysis of the multiple logistic regression met the Hosmer and Lemeshow criteria (1989), where the good fit of the proposed final model can be verified by the non-significant difference between the predicted and observed probabilities. The significant variables included were part of the model's fit, according to the HOSMER-LEMESHOW chi-square (p<0.05).

The study was submitted to the Research Ethics Committee of the State University of Ceará and the Assis Chateubriand Maternity School, and received a favourable opinion, protocol no. 030/12, issued on 31 July 2012. The research therefore complied with Resolution 466/2012 (BRASIL, 2012).

RESULTS

The results of this study are presented according to the hierarchical model for the study of neonatal death (outcome), with descriptive and inferential analysis of the data (Block 01 and Block 02).

Table 01 shows the distal level variables relating to the neonatal death outcome and the mother's socioeconomic and demographic characteristics.

Table 01. Unadjusted distal risk factors for neonatal mortality, according to mothers' socioeconomic and demographic characteristics, Fortaleza, CE, BR, 2009 and 2010.

VARIABLES	CASE n(=153)	%	CONTROL n(=464)	%	Unadjusted OR	95% CI	P
Years of study							
>4	134	87,58	435	93,75	1,0		
<4	19	12,42	29	6,25	2,13	1,15; 3,92 0	0,01
Marital status							
Live together	40	26,14	103	22,20	1,0		
Not living together	113	73,86	361	77,80	0,8	0,52; 1,22	0,31
*Work							
No	77	50,33	224	64,93	1,0		
Yes	76	49,67	121	35,07	1,83	1,23; 2,70	<0,001

95% CI: 95% confidence interval; OR: odds ratio.

In this block, the majority of mothers had four or more years of schooling, both in cases 134 (87.58%) and controls 435 (93.75%), with (OR=2.13; CI 1.15;3.92), not living together with their partner 113 (73.86%) in cases and 361 (77.80%) in controls, with (OR=0.8; CI 0.52;1.22) and not working 77 (50.33%) cases and 224 (64.93%)

controls, with (OR=1.83; CI 1.23;2.70).

In the univariate analysis, the variables years of schooling and working were associated (p<0.20) with the outcome. Mothers who studied for less than four years were 2.1 times more likely to have their children die, while working mothers were 1.8 times more likely to reach the outcome. The marital status variable was not associated with the outcome (p >0.20).

Table 02: Intermediate risk factors I, unadjusted for neonatal mortality, according to maternal characteristics, Fortaleza, CE, BR, 2009 and 2010.

	CASE		CONTROL				
VARIABLES	N=15 3	%	N=46 4	%	Unadjust ed OR	95% CI	P
Maternal age (years)							
5 20	94	61,44	308	66,38	1,0		
< 20	59	38,56	156	33,62	1,24	0,84; 1,81	0,27
Gestational age (weeks)							
>37	21	13,73	392	84,48	1,0		
< 37	132	86,27	72	15,52	34,2	17,15; 68,26	<0,001
Type of pregnancy							
Unique	136	88,89	441	95,04	1,0		
Multiple	17	11,11	23	4,96	2,39	1,23; 4,63	<0,001
Number of previous pregnancies							
3 or more	49	32,03	134	28,88	1,0		
<2	104	67,97	330	71,12	0,86	0,58; 1,28	0,46
Number of births							
Primipara	58	37,91	223	48,06	1,0		
Multiparous	95	62,09	241	51,94	1,52	1,04; 2,20	0,03
Number of miscarriages							
None	114	74,51	359	77,37	1,0		
> 1	39	25,49	105	22,63	1,16	0,76; 1,78	0,46
Urinary Tract Infection							
No	129	84,31	398	85,78	1,0		
Yes	24	15,69	66	14,22	1,12	0,67; 1,86	0,65
HAS							
No	135	88,24	410	88,36	1,0		
Yes	18	11,76	54	11,64	1,01	0,57; 1,78	0,96
Drug use							
No	99	86,09	410	91,11	1,0		
Yes	16	13,91	14	8,89	1,65	0,88; 3,08	0,10
Smoking during pregnancy							
No	142	92,81	435	93,75	1,0		
Yes	11	7,19	29	6,25	1,16	0,56; 2,39	0,68

Alcohol during pregnancy							
No	143	93,46	444	95,69	1,0		
Yes	10	6,54	20	4,31	1,55	0,70; 3,40	0,26
Other drugs							
No	151	98,69	460	99,14	1,0		
Yes	2	1,31	4	0,86	1,52	0,27; 8,41	0,62

95% CI: 95% confidence interval; OR: odds ratio.

Table 02 shows maternal characteristics. The mean maternal age was 25.13 years, with a standard deviation of 8.68 years. Most mothers were aged 20 or over, both in the 94 cases (61.44%) and in the 308 controls (66.38%) (OR=1.24; CI 0.84; 1.81).

The univariate analysis in Table 02 revealed an association only between the gestational age and type of pregnancy variables ($p<0.20$). Gestational age of less than 37 weeks was 34.2 times more likely (OR) to lead to neonatal death. Multiple gestation was also more likely to trigger the outcome (OR=2.39). Multiparity was also associated ($p=0.02$). The other variables showed no association ($p>0.20$).

The inferential analysis revealed that gestational age < 37 weeks was higher in 132 cases (86.27%); in the controls, gestational age > 37 weeks was predominant in 392 (84.48%), with a mean of 35.65 gestational weeks, with a standard deviation of 5.41 gestational weeks and (OR=34.2; CI 17.15; 68.26). The single pregnancy type in cases and controls prevailed with 136 (88.89%) and 441 (95.04%), respectively, (OR=2.39; CI 1.23; 4.63).

The mean number of pregnancies was 2.21, with a standard deviation of 1.56 pregnancies, with a predominance of pregnancies < 2, in 104 cases (67.97 per cent) and 330 controls (71.12 per cent) (OR=0.86; CI 0.58; 1.28). All the following variables were predominant in cases and controls. Multiparous women, cases 95 (62.09%) and controls 241 (51.94%) (OR=1.52; CI 1.04; 2.20), those who had not had an abortion, cases 114 (74.51%) and controls 359 (77.37%) (OR=1.16; CI 0.76; 1.78), those without urinary tract infection, cases 129 (84.31%) and controls 398 (85.78%) and (OR=1.12; CI 0.67; 1.86) and systemic arterial hypertension, cases 135 (88.24%) and controls 410 (88.36%) (OR=1.01; CI 0.57; 1.78).

Drug use during pregnancy was higher in 16 cases (13.91%) than in 14 controls (8.89%) (OR=1.65; CI 0.88; 3.08). As for the type of drug used (smoking, alcohol and other drugs), there was also a predominance in cases.

Women who did not smoke had 142 cases (92.81%) and 435 controls (93.75%) (OR=1.16; CI 0.56; 2.39); those who did not use alcohol, cases

143 (93.46%) and controls 444 (95.69%) (OR=1.55; CI 0.70; 3.40); and did not use other drugs, cases 151 (98.69%) and controls 460 (99.14%) (OR=1.52; CI 0.27; 8.41); were predominant in the study.

DISCUSSION

The use of secondary data in research into risk factors for infant mortality is important, but it can reveal some flaws in hospital records. This can be considered a limitation of the study, as some of the information may not be complete, either because it was not recorded or because it was not given due importance by the professionals who recorded it.

The medical records should contain precise and detailed information on all the care provided to pregnant women, postpartum women and newborns, as well as the patients' prenatal and clinical history. However, what we realised was that a lot of the information was incomplete, leaving a gap in the patients' clinical history.

In addition to medical records, information from the SINASC and SIM health systems, both of which are used throughout the country, should be highlighted. These should be the most reliable sources of information on births and deaths, generating real indicators and making a major contribution to public health. Studying the profile of births and deaths is fundamental for drawing up well-targeted public policies. The data collection technique used in this research revealed and confirmed the incompleteness of the databases generated from the national information systems SINASC and SIM.

The infant deaths presented in this study indicate that the neonatal component contributes the highest percentage of infant mortality. This finding corroborates the results found in other studies. Risso and **Nascimento (2011), in their study "Risk factors for neonatal death obtained by the multivariate Cox regression model", point to** the fall in infant mortality rates, indicating the concentration of deaths in the neonatal period, remaining significantly high compared to the lower post-neonatal mortality rates; in which the majority of neonatal deaths occurred in the early neonatal component.

Silva et al. (2012), in their study on infant mortality carried out in the city of Pelotas, RS, found that around 70% of infant deaths occurred in the neonatal period, and of these, approximately 68% occurred before 7 days of life. Carneiro et al. (2012), in their study carried out in the north of Minas Gerais, aimed to identify the factors associated with the mortality of very low birth weight newborns admitted to a reference Neonatal Intensive Care Unit. The authors show the importance of the neonatal component in the constitution of infant mortality, generating studies and innovations in research into the causes and determinants of death in this period.

With regard to the maternal schooling variable, it was noted that the majority of mothers, in both cases and controls, had studied for four years or more; mothers who had studied for less than four years were at twice the risk of neonatal deaths. Similar results are cited by Jobim and Aerts (2008) in their study on preventable infant mortality and associated factors in Porto Alegre, RS, where they studied 1,139 infant deaths for which a Death Certificate (DC) was issued. The results showed that the majority of mothers, 514 (45.1%), had between four and seven years of schooling.

This demonstrates the improvement in socio-economic conditions that has been reflected in various aspects of society; the increase in maternal schooling allows women to take a new look at their health and that of their families. Education is fundamental for people to take responsibility for their health/disease process. Thus, mothers who had more years of schooling showed greater protection against neonatal death.

The mothers' marital status is also described in this study, in which the majority of them do not live with their partner. Caputo and Bordin (2008), in a study of 408 adolescents in a municipality in São Paulo, found that the majority of pregnant women did not live with their boyfriend or husband 61 (61%), corroborating the findings of this study.

Living or not living with a partner may be a reflection of the new status of women in society with greater independence; it may also be related to new family configurations, with marital relationships that are losing their husband-wife characteristics, demonstrating the fragility of the bond between people. Today, the choice of pregnancy no longer depends on the marital situation experienced by the woman.

In this sense, according to Coelho et al, (2012), in their study "Association between unplanned pregnancy and the socioeconomic context of women in a Family Health Strategy area", these researchers found that pregnancy from the perspective of reproductive rights and the choice of a pregnancy passing through the plane of rationality, results from the exercise of a woman's autonomy and reproductive freedom. Thus, pregnancy resulting from a process in which there was no conscious decision by the woman or the couple for it to occur is considered to be unplanned.

When the mothers' work was analysed, the majority did not work. This was protective for neonatal death. Mothers who worked had a 1.83 higher risk of neonatal death. Corroborating these results, Nascimento et al. (2012), in their study on the determinants of neonatal mortality in Fortaleza, Ceará, found that in both cases and controls, most mothers did not work during pregnancy and had no occupation.

Some possibilities can be put forward to explain this protective factor for neonatal death. Women who don't work may have more time to monitor their pregnancy, and may also have a lower risk of pregnancy due to risky work activities.

Maternal age from 20 years onwards could mean a reduction in teenage pregnancies. These findings are corroborated by Domingues et al. (2012), in a study carried out in Rio de Janeiro, which found that pregnant women were predominantly aged between 20 and 34. (2011), on the contextual determinants of neonatal mortality in Rio Grande do Sul, the findings were similar, with approximately 70 per cent of women in this age group.

The association between infant mortality and twinning has been reported by several authors. Twinning is considered an important risk factor for infant mortality, as this condition is often related to low birth weight and lower gestational age. Therefore, live births from single pregnancies were less likely to die. It is worth pointing out that premature live births and low birth weight are more frequent in multiple pregnancies (MARAN and UCHIMURA, 2008).

Women who had two or fewer pregnancies were predominant in both cases and controls. Poles and Parada (2002) found **different results in their study on "Infant mortality in a municipality** in the interior of the state of São Paulo", which **found** that mortality was higher in the case of mothers who had more pregnancies, i.e. in large multiparous women.

Hernandez et al. (2011), in their study analysing trends in infant mortality rates and their risk factors in the city of Porto Alegre, Rio Grande do Sul, highlighted the downward trend in multiparity. However, the results of this study revealed that women who have only had one child are still in the minority, although they tend to be closer to women who have had more than one birth; multiparous women had an increased risk of 1.52.

As for the number of miscarriages, mothers who had no miscarriages prevailed.

However, among mothers who had at least one abortion, the prevalence was in the case group. Oliveira, Gama and Silva (2010), in a study carried out in the municipality of Rio de Janeiro, found no statistical association between abortion and infant death.

Another factor that must be taken into account is the woman's medical history, existing illnesses or those acquired during pregnancy.

Urinary tract infection (UTI) is a very common clinical manifestation in women, and even more so in pregnant women, where the presence of the disease may not represent a high risk, but if it is not treated, or is treated inadequately, it can cause gestational risks, such as premature labour or even cause infections in the newborn. Early diagnosis during prenatal care is therefore essential for effective treatment. Duarte et al. (2008), in their study on urinary infection in pregnancy, highlighted the main gestational complications, such as labour and preterm delivery, low birth weight, premature rupture of amniotic membranes, intrauterine growth restriction, cerebral palsy/mental retardation and perinatal death.

In this study, the results only refer to the presence or absence of infection during pregnancy, and do not allow for an analysis of treatment. This can be considered a limitation of the study using secondary data, since the information on UTI treatment was not present in the medical records. The presence of UTI represented an increased risk of 1.12 compared to non-infection.

Although the presence of UTI did not represent the majority of the sample studied, due to its clinical importance, it should not be disregarded, as it can lead to maternal complications, such as pre-term labour and sepsis. UTI can lead to perinatal complications, low birth weight, intrauterine growth restriction and even infant death (CALEGARI et al., 2012).

Systemic arterial hypertension (SAH) is another disease of great importance when monitoring pregnant women, because depending on how it **develops, it can be fatal for mothers and newborns.** Pregnant **women with** decompensated **hypertension** can develop into pre-eclampsia and eclampsia.

In this study, information was collected from medical records on the registration of SAH. In the medical records studied, the majority of the sample did not have this information, which was interpreted as not having the disease. Among those who had a record of hypertension, the difference between cases and controls was insignificant.

The literature points to hypertension as the main cause of maternal death, and it can also influence infant mortality, with foetal complications, including prematurity and low birth weight. Early diagnosis, monitoring and treatment are essential to avoid maternal and foetal complications (FREIRE; TEDOLDI, 2009).

According to Santos et al (2009), in their study "Risk factors for pregnancy-specific hypertensive syndrome**",** hypertensive **disorders are** the most important complications during the pregnancy-puerperal period, contributing significantly to both maternal and foetal morbidity and mortality.

Another important factor that has been observed in recent years is the increase in drug use among men and women, with women being the biggest concern. The consumption of alcohol, tobacco and other drugs is considered a public health problem, with physical and social repercussions.

In this study, drug use was not prevalent, but there was an increased risk of neonatal death.

The use of drugs is something that can be found in hospital records, but due to the stigma that exists in society, women often don't report the use of these substances. According to Sousa, Santos and Oliveira (2012), pregnant women may report less alcohol consumption or deny it in order to avoid possible reprimand and disapproval from health professionals.

Health professionals must therefore be sensitised to this reality, avoiding embarrassing women and gaining their trust in the search for reliable information.

Among the drugs with the most records, smoking was the most common. This can be explained by the fact that it is not considered an illicit drug, although its use can lead to maternal and foetal complications. Reggiani et al., (2004), show that approximately 25% of pregnant women use tobacco, surpassing the use of illicit drugs.

In 2004, the World Health Organisation (WHO) estimated that 12% of the world's adult female population were smokers. Schoeps et al. (2007), in their study on "Risk factors for early neonatal mortality", did not find cigarette consumption to be the majority, but with data close to the first quintile and quartile for cases and controls respectively.

Tobacco use during pregnancy has implications for maternal and foetal health. There are so many harmful effects on foetal health that it can be said that the foetus is a true active smoker (BASTOS; BORNIA, 2009).

The literature presents exposure to drugs during pregnancy as a risk factor for infant death, mainly due to the teratogenic characteristics of licit and illicit drugs. Even though there is no significant association with the outcome, drug use cannot be ignored as a risk. Nascimento et al. (2012) corroborated these findings and found no statistical association between drug use and infant death.

The treatment of women who use drugs should increasingly be included in public health policies, with a view to their recovery and avoiding maternal and foetal risks.

It should be emphasised that drug use during pregnancy is a risk factor that can be avoided if prenatal care is carried out. Hence the importance that should be attached to prenatal care, as good monitoring favours a safer pregnancy, thereby avoiding maternal and foetal risks.

CONCLUSION

Most mothers had four years or more of schooling, did not live with a partner and did not work. With regard to the variables relating to maternal characteristics; the majority of mothers were aged 20 or over, gestational age of less than 37 weeks was prevalent in neonatal deaths and 37 weeks or over was prevalent in survivors of the neonatal period; the majority of mothers had a single pregnancy, two or fewer pregnancies, more than two births, no abortions and did not use drugs during pregnancy.

The results of this study point mainly to the importance of prenatal care in monitoring pregnant women. This is when various risks can be eliminated or controlled. Even though it did not appear in the final model, prenatal care is a variable that is strongly linked to a reduction in gestational and neonatal risks.

Some recommendations should be considered as effective public health policy actions, such as: expanding the women's health care network, improving women's access to prenatal care, whether they are at risk or not, providing quality care by carrying out the tests recommended by the Ministry of Health in good time, guaranteeing a referral maternity hospital for childbirth, avoiding women's pilgrimage.

REFERENCES

BASTOS, M.S.; BORNIA, E.C.S. **Use of nicotine and/or cocaine during pregnancy and its consequences on foetal and neonatal development**. VI Encontro Internacional de Produção Científica Cesumar 27 to 30 October 2009. ISBN 978-85-61091-05-7.

BORGES, J.A.M. **Study of gestational drug addiction and neonatal death**. Fortaleza, 2012. 91f. Dissertation (Master's in Public Health) - Health Sciences Centre, State University of Ceará, 2012.

BRAZIL. Ministry of Health. National Health Council. Resolution 466/12. **Provides guidelines and regulatory standards for research involving human beings**. Brasília: National Health Council, 2012.

BRAZIL. Ministry of Health. Health Care Secretariat. Department of Programme and Strategic Actions. **Newborn health care**: a guide for health professionals. Brasília: Ministry of Health, 2011.
Available at <http://www.redeblh.fiocruz.br/media/arn v1.pdf> Accessed 25 Jun 2016.

BRAZIL. Ministry of Health. Health Surveillance Secretariat. Health Care Secretariat. **Manual for the surveillance of infant and foetal death and the Committee for the Prevention of Infant and Foetal Death**. 2. ed. Brasília: Ministry of Health, 2009. Available at
<http://bvsms.saude.gov.br/bvs/publicacoes/manual obito infantil fetal 2ed.pd f>
Accessed 24 Jun 2016.

CALEGARI, S.S.; et al. Results of two treatment regimens for pyelonephritis during pregnancy and correlation with pregnancy outcome.
Brazilian Journal of Gynaecology and Obstetrics, v.34, n.8, p.369-375, 2012.

CAPUTO, V.G.; BORDIN, I.A. Pregnancy in adolescence and frequent use of alcohol and drugs in the family context. **Revista de Saúde Pública**, v.42, n.3, p.402-410, 2008.

CARNEIRO, J.A.; et al. Risk factors for mortality of very low birth weight infants in the Neonatal Intensive Care Unit. **Revista Paulista de Pediatria**, v.30, n.3, p.369-376, 2012.

CARRANZA, D.V.V.; PEDRÃO, L.J. Personal satisfaction of the drug-addicted adolescent in the family environment during the treatment phase at a

institute of mental health. **Revista Latino-Americana de Enfermagem**, v.13, special edition, p.836-844, 2005.

CARLINI, E.A.; GALDURÓZ, J.C.F.; NOTO, A.R.; NAPPO, S.A.**I Household survey on the use of psychotropic drugs in Brazil: a study involving the 107 largest cities in the country**. 2001. São Paulo (SP): Brazilian Centre for Information on Psychotropic Drugs. UNIFESP - Federal University of São Paulo, 2002.

CARLINI, E.A. SUPERVISOR. **II Household survey on the use of psychotropic drugs in Brazil: a study involving the 108 largest cities in the country**. 2005. São Paulo (SP): CEBRID, UNIFESP - Federal University of São Paulo, 2006.

COELHO, E.A.C.; et al. Association between unplanned pregnancy and the socioeconomic context of women in a Family Health Strategy area. **Acta Paul Enferm**, v.25, n.3, p.415-422, 2012.

DANTAS, S.L.D.; et al. Use of the linkage method to identify risk factors associated with infant mortality: an integrative literature review. **Ciência & Saúde Coletiva**, v.19, n.7, p.2095-2104, 2014.

DOMINGUES, R.M.S.M.; et al. Evaluation of the adequacy of prenatal care in the SUS network of the Municipality of Rio de Janeiro, Brazil. **Cadernos de Saúde Pública**, v.28, n.3, p.425-437, 2012.

DUARTE, G.; et al. Urinary infection in pregnancy. **Revista Brasileira de Ginecologia e Obstetrícia**, v.30, n.2, p.93-100, 2008.

FREIRE, C.M.V.; TEDOLDI, C.L. Hypertension in pregnancy. **Arquivos Brasileiros de Cardiologia**, v.93, n.6, p.110-178, 2009.

GAIVA, M.A.M.; BITTENCOURT, R.M.; FUJIMORI, E. Early and late neonatal death: profile of mothers and newborns. **Revista Gaúcha de Enfermagem**, v.34, n.4, p.91-97, 2013a.

GAIVA, M.A.M.; FUJIMORI, E.; SATO, A.P.S. Neonatal mortality in low birth weight infants. **Revista da Escola de Enfermagem USP**, v.48, n.5, p.778-786, 2014.

HERNANDEZ, A.R.; et al. Trend analysis of infant mortality rates and their risk factors in the city of Porto Alegre, Rio Grande do Sul, Brazil, from 1996 to 2008. **Cadernos de Saúde Pública**, v.27, n.11, p.2188-2196, 2011.

HOSMER, D.W.; LEMESHOW, S. **Applied logistic regression**. New York: John Wiley & Sons, 1989.

JOBIM, R., AERTS D. Preventable infant mortality and associated factors in Porto Alegre, Rio Grande do Sul, Brazil, 2000-2003. **Cadernos de Saúde Pública**, v.24, n.1, p.179-189, 2008.

LIMA, S., CARVALHO, M.L., VASCONCELOS, A.G.G. Proposal for a hierarchical model applied to the investigation of risk factors for neonatal infant death. **Cadernos de Saúde Pública**, v.24, n.8, p.1910-1916, 2008.

MENDES, K.G.; OLINTO, M.T.A.; COSTA, J.S.D. Case-control study on infant mortality in Southern Brazil. **Revista de Saúde Pública**, v.40, n.2, p.240-248, 2006.

MARAM, E.; UCHIMURA, T.T. Neonatal mortality: risk factors in a municipality in southern Brazil**. Revista Eletrônica de Enfermagem**, v.10, n.1, p.29-38, 2008.

NASCIMENTO, R.M.; et al. Determinants of neonatal mortality: a case-control study in Fortaleza, Ceará, Brazil. **Cadernos de Saúde Pública**, v.28, n.3, p.559-572, 2012.

OLIVEIRA, E.F.V.; GAMA, S.G.N.G.; SILVA, C.M.F.P. Teenage pregnancy and other risk factors for foetal and infant mortality in the municipality of Rio de Janeiro, Brazil. **Cadernos de Saúde Pública**, v.26, n.3, p.567-578, 2010.

PINHEIRO, S.N.; LAPREGA, M.R.; FURTADO, E.F. Morbidade psiquiátrica e uso de álcool em gestantes usuárias do Sistema Único de Saúde. **Revista de Saúde Pública**, v.39, n.4, p.593-598, 2005.

POLES, K.; PARADA, C.M.G. L. Infant mortality in a municipality in the interior of the State of São Paulo. **Revista da Escola de Enfermagem USP**, v.36, n.1, p.10-17,

2002.

REGGIANI, C.P.D.; et al. Fetal and Neonatal Effects of Nicotine and **Crack** Use **During Pregnancy. Brazilian Journal of Medicine**, v.87, s/n, p.46-49, 2004.

RISSO, S.P.; NASCIMENTO, L.F.C. Risk factors for death in a neonatal intensive care unit, using the survival analysis technique. **Revista Brasileira de Terapia Intensiva**, v.22, n.1, p.19-26, 2010.

RUTSTEIN, D.D.; et al. Measuring the quality of medical care: a clinical method. **N Engl J Med**, v.2, n.94, p.582-588, 1976.

REGO, M.A.V. Case-control studies: a brief review. **Gazeta Médica da Bahia**, v.79, n.1, p.101-110, 2010.

SANTOS, Z.M.S.A.; et al. Risk factors for pregnancy-specific hypertensive syndrome. **Revista Brasileira em Promoção da Saúde**, v.22, n.1, p.48-54, 2009.

SMS - TABNET, Fortaleza. Epidemiological Surveillance Cell. Available at: <www.saudefortaleza.ce.gov.br>. Accessed on: 30 August 2011.

SILVA, V.L.S.; et al. Infant mortality in the city of Pelotas, state of Rio Grande do Sul, Brazil, in the period 2005-2008: use of death investigation in the analysis of preventable causes. **Epidemiologia e Serviços de Saúde**, v.21, n.2, p.265-274, 2012.

SOUZA, L.H.R.F.; SANTOS, M.C.; OLIVEIRA, L.C.M. Pattern of alcohol consumption in pregnant women treated at a public university hospital and associated risk factors. **Revista Brasileira de Ginecologia e Obstetrícia**, v.34, n.7, p.296-303, 2012.

SCHOEPS, D.; et al. Risk Factors for Early Neonatal Mortality. **Revista de Saúde Pública**, v.41, n.6, p.1013-1022, 2007.

UNITED NATIONS OFFICE ON DRUGS AND CRIME. **World Drug Programme, 2010**. Brasilia: UNODC Brazil and Southern Cone, 2010. Available at: <http://www.unodc.org/brazil/pt/prevencao_drogas.html>. Accessed on: 09 January 2012.

VICTORA, C.G.; et al. The role of conceptual frameworks in epidemiological analysis: a hierarchical approach. **International Journal of Epidemiology**, v.26, n.1, p.224-227, 1997.

ZANINI, R.R.; et al. Contextual determinants of neonatal mortality in Rio Grande do Sul using two analysis models. **Revista de Saúde Publica**, v.45, n.1, p.79-89, 2011.

CHAPTER 4

FACTORS INVOLVED IN MORBIDITY AND MORTALITY DUE TO VERTICAL TRANSMISSION OF SYPHILIS IN A CAPITAL CITY IN NORTHEASTERN BRAZIL

Francisca Cláudia Monteiro Almeida

Francisco José Maia Pinto

Radmila Alves Alencar Viana

Jéssica Karen de Oliveira Maia

Priscila Nunes Costa Travassos

Dandhara Kathleen Monteiro Vaz

Daniele Silva de Oliveira

INTRODUCTION

As a result of our country's social and health reality, deaths continue to occur due to preventable diseases, through health actions and services, including prenatal care, childbirth and newborn care. Regardless of the expansion of prenatal care, the incidence of congenital syphilis remains high, indicating an unfavourable situation regarding the quality of prenatal care (BRASIL, 2013).

Syphilis is an infectious disease caused by a gram-negative bacterium called Treponema pallidum (MAGALHÃES et al., 2013). Relatively 2 million pregnant women in the world are infected each year due to a lack of diagnosis and when the infection is confirmed, early treatment does not occur or is neglected. Approximately 50% of women with untreated syphilis transmit the infection to their foetus, causing adverse outcomes (i.e. stillbirth, neonatal death, prematurity, low birth weight, or infant with congenital infection), comprising an estimated 440,000 perinatal deaths per year (WHO, 2011).

According to the World Health Organisation (WHO), 1 million new cases of syphilis in pregnant women are expected every year. In Brazil, 21,382 new cases were detected in pregnant women in 2013 (BRASIL, 2015). Its high prevalence, 1.9 per cent for the Northeast region, is due to many factors, including low or non-adherence to prenatal care, incomplete or inadequate treatment of pregnant women and their partners, and underreporting of cases (COSTA et al., 2013).

The state of Ceará has the second highest rate in the country (7.1 per 1,000 live births), second only to Rio de Janeiro (9.8 per 100 live births). By September 2013, according to the epidemiological report, 511 cases had been notified and investigated, representing an incidence rate of 6.9/1000 live births (CEARÁ, 2013).

It is known that prenatal care is of great importance for identifying new cases and, above all, for maintaining treatment and serological monitoring of pregnant women and their partners, preventing reinfection (BRASIL, 2012; COSTA et al., 2013).

The importance of this research is due to the discussion on the control of syphilis in pregnant women during prenatal care, because when carried out properly, it can prevent negative outcomes for the mother-child binomial.

Faced with the magnitude of the problem of reducing the number of cases and the incidence of gestational syphilis, professionals came up with the idea of looking for ways to improve public policies to help reduce the prevalence of syphilis and its maternal and child complications.

This study is an excerpt from Almeida's dissertation (2012) and aimed to analyse the factors involved in the morbidity and mortality of vertical transmission of syphilis associated with gestational outcome in reference maternity hospitals in Fortaleza, Ceará - Brazil.

METHODS

A cross-sectional study, with a descriptive and analytical approach, carried out in three public maternity hospitals, representative of the federal, state and municipal spheres in the municipality of Fortaleza - CE, between May and October 2012, one year after the implementation of the Stork Network in the state.

The sample consisted of 119 women admitted to one of the three public maternity hospitals due to pregnancy loss with positive VDRL at the time of hospital admission for labour/curettage. Those in a clinical mental state that made it impossible to answer the questionnaire at the time of collection were excluded, as were those who did not live in Fortaleza.

The outcome variable was gestational loss dichotomised as yes or no and the explanatory variables were: sociodemographic, gynaecological and obstetric, current pregnancy, partner and conceptus.

Data collection was based on secondary data, with information gathered from medical records, prenatal care cards and SINAN (Information System for Notifiable Diseases) forms relating to congenital syphilis. Primary information was obtained using a semi-structured form from the women identified in the hospital epidemiology centres (NUHEP) and who were in the puerperium ward.

Initially, in the univariate model (crude analysis), association tests were carried out between the outcome variable and the explanatory variables, using Pearson's chi-square or Monte Carlo tests, at a 5% significance level.

In the adjusted analysis, only the explanatory variables that showed p<0.20 in the crude analysis were considered for participation in the model and only those that were significant with p<5% were considered to remain in the final model, according to Victora et al. (1997).

Poisson regression with robust variance was used as an adjusted estimate of PR (Barros & Hirakata, 2003). This model should be used to estimate PR per point and per interval in cross-sectional studies with binary outcomes (COUTINHO; SCARZUFCA; MENENZES, 2008).

The data was tabulated in the EXCEL programme and processed in Predictive Analytics Software For Windows (PASW), version 17.0.

The study was submitted to the Research Ethics Committee of the State University of Ceará (UECE), approved under protocol number 16549, and was also scrutinised by the committees of the hospitals studied.

RESULTS

It was found that the majority of pregnant women, 83 (69.8%), had prenatal care, attended appointments at the basic health unit, 66 (79.5%) and were seen by a doctor and nurse, 55 (66.3%), with between 1 and 5 appointments during pregnancy, 50 (60.2%). Although it is not recommended by the Ministry of Health, the majority of pregnant women, 45 (54.2%), started prenatal care in the second trimester. Furthermore, the diagnosis of syphilis was only detected during prenatal care, 67(53.6%) and only 34(41.0%) of them completed treatment at this stage. There was no care taken to use condoms, even after the disease was discovered 56(82.4%). Also, the partner rejected drug therapy or didn't turn up 101(84.9%), while for pregnant women, treatment was considered inadequate 86(72.3%), leading to miscarriage or stillbirth in 18(15.1%) of the women. The average number of consultations was approximately 5, with a standard deviation of 2 (TABLE 1).

Table 1: Distribution of women according to the characteristics of their current pregnancy. Fortaleza, CE, 2012

Variables	Mean (SD)	n	%
Had prenatal care (n=119)			
No		36	30,2
Yes		83	69,8
Prenatal site (n=83)			
USB		66	79,5
Hospital		15	2,4
Agreement		0,2	18,1
Professional who carried out the PN (n=83)			
Doctor/nurse		55	66,3
Doctor		23	27,7
Don't know		05	6,0
No. of consultations (n=83)	4,8(2,0)		
1 a 5		50	60,2
6 a 10		33	39,8
Start of PN (n=83)			
1st quarter		26	31,3
2nd quarter		45	54,2
3rd quarter		12	14,5
Syphilis diagnosis			
Prenatal care		67	53,6
Childbirth/curettage		52	43,7
Post-diagnosis condom (n=68)			
No		56	82,4
Yes		12	17,6
VDRL 1st trimester (n=26)			
Realised		22	84,6
Not realised		04	15,4
VDRL 2nd trimester (n=83)			
Realised		60	72,3
Not realised/no information		23	27,7
Monthly VDRL (n=83)			
Realised		40	48,2
Not realised/no information		43	51,8
Concomitant partner treatment (n=119)			
No		18	15,1
Yes/no information		101	84,9
Treatment for syphilis (n=119)			
Suitable		33	27,7
Inadequate		86	72,3
Outcome of pregnancy (n=119)			
Born alive		101	84,9
Abortion/miscarriage		18	15,1

There was a predominance of items referring to lack of interest in seeking follow-up 14 (38.9%), followed by the use of alcohol and/or other drugs 13 (36.1%), the most frequent being crack (GRAPH 1).

Among the reasons given by the women for not **treating their partner, "the partner's non-attendance or refusal to undergo treatment" was simply the most prominent, 18 (29.5%)** (GRAPH 2).

In the univariate model relating the outcome of pregnancy loss to the explanatory variables (sociodemographic, gynaecological and obstetric), the following were identified as statistically significant at the 5% level: marital status (p=0.013), occupation (p=0.005) and history of abortion (p<0.001). At the borderline, family income in minimum wages was indicated (p=0.057), and was therefore disregarded in the study. In other words, the chance of pregnancy loss is: approximately 4 times for those not living in a conjugal union and more than 5 times for those with a history of miscarriage (TABLE 2).

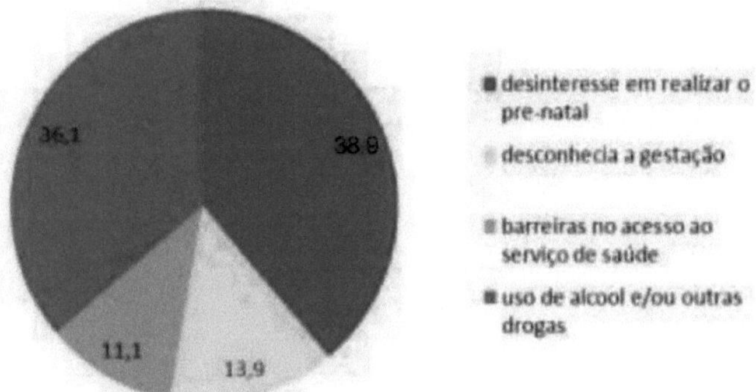

Graph 1: Reasons given by women for not having prenatal care. Fortaleza-CE, 2012

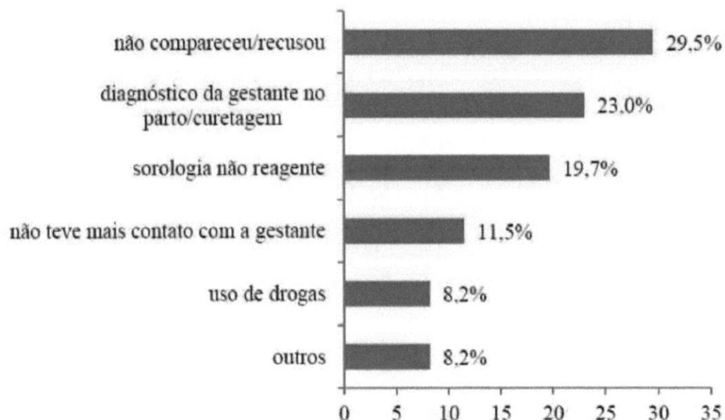

Graph 2: Reasons for not treating partner concomitantly. Fortaleza, CE, 2012

Table 2: Univariate analysis of the gestational loss outcome with sociodemographic, gynaecological and obstetric characteristics. Fortaleza, CE, 2012. (continued)

Variables	Gestational loss				Unadjusted PR	95% CI	Value of p
	Yes n	%	No N	%			
Mother's age in years							
< 20 years	6	20,0	24	80,0	1,48	0,61 ; 3,61	0,384
> 20 years	12	13,5	77	86,5			
Skin colour							
Brown/black	17	15,2	95	84,8	1,06	0,16 ; 6,87	0,949
White	1	14,3	6	85,7			
Years of study							
Up to 9 years old	15	14,7	87	85,3	0,83	0,27 ; 2,58	0,751
Over 9 years old	3	17,6	14	82,4			
Marital status							
They don't live together	14	24,6	43	75,4	3,81	1,33 ; 10,89	**0,013**
They live together	4	6,5	58	93,5			
Occupation							
Unpaid	7	8,5	75	91,5	0,29	0,12 ; 0,68	**0,005**
Paid	11	29,7	26	70,3			
Family income in minimum wages							
< 1	1	2,9	33	97,1	0,15	0,02 ; 1,06	0,057
> 1	17	20,0	68	80,0			
Start of sexual activity in years							
10 to 13 years	10	16,4	51	83,6	1,19	0,50 ; 2,80	0,693
14 to 20 years	8	13,8	50	86,2			
No. of partners in the last year							
1	11	14,9	63	85,1	0,96	0,40 ; 2,29	0,919
2 or more	7	15,6	38	84,4			
Unique partner at the moment							
No	3	13,0	20	87,0	0,98	0,30 ; 3,18	0,971
Yes	12	13,3	78	86,7			
Condom use							
Sometimes	7	12,3	50	87,7	1,44	0,60 ; 3,47	0,411
Never	11	17,7	51	82,3			
History of syphilis							
No	0	0,0	14	100,0	1,44	0,60 ; 3,47	0,411
Yes	10	12,2	72	87,8	1		
History of another STD							
No	4	18,2	18	81,8	1,82	0,60;5,485,48	0,288
Yes	8	10,0	72	90,0	1		
No. of pregnancies							

1	7	20,6	27	79,4	1,59	0,67	3,76	0,290
2 or more	11	12,9	74	87,1	1			
History of abortion								
Yes	12	36,4	21	63,6	5,21	2,13	12,74	**<0,001**
No	6	7,0	80	93,0	1			
History of foetal death								
Yes	3	20,0	12	80,0	1,39	0,45	4,23	0,566
No	15	14,4	89	85,6	1			
History of premature labour								
Yes	4	12,1	29	87,9	0,74	0,26	2,10	0,577
No	14	16,3	72	83,7	1			

Source: Research data

In the univariate model for the outcome of pregnancy loss with the explanatory variables (current pregnancy, partner and conceptus), the following were identified as statistically significant at the 5% level: Prenatal care (p<0.001), Time with partner in years (p=0.018), Gestational age (p=0.001) and Birth weight in grams (p=0.011). In other words, the chance of pregnancy loss is: more than 8 times for those who don't have prenatal care; more than 4 times when the partner has been living with them for less than 2 years and approximately 13 times when the women have a gestational age of less than 37 weeks (TABLE 3).

Table 3: Univariate analysis of the gestational loss outcome with the characteristics of the current pregnancy, partner and conceptus. Fortaleza, CE, 2012

	Gestational loss						
	Yes		No				
Variables	**n**	**%**	**N**	**%**	**Unadjusted PR**	**95% CI**	**p-value**
Had prenatal care							
No	14	38,9	22	61,1	8,07	2,85 ; 22,83	**<0,001**
Yes	4	4,8	79	95,2	1		
No. of enquiries							
less than 6	3	6,0	47	94,0	1,98	0,22 ; 18,23	0,546
6 or more	1	3,0	32	97,0	1		
Start of the NP							
1st quarter	3	5,3	54	94,7	1,37	0,15 12,54	0,781
2nd or 3rd trimester	1	3,8	25	96,2	1		
VDRL 3rd trimester (n=83)							
Not realised/no information	3	13,0	20	87,0	7,83	0,86 71,45	0,068
Realised	1	1,7	59	98,3	1		
Monthly VDRL (n=83)							
Not realised/no information	3	7,0	40	93,0	2,79	0,30 25,74	0,365
Realised	1	2,5	39	97,5	1		

Treatment for syphilis								
Inadequate	17	19,8	69	80,2	6,52	0,90	47,08	0,063
Suitable	1	3,0	32	97,0	1			
Time with partner in years								
Less than 2	9	23,1	30	76,9	4,46	1,29	15,45	**0,018**
2 or more	3	5,2	55	94,8	1			
Partner treatment								
No/no information	17	16,8	84	83,2	3,03	0,43	21,37	0,266
Yes	1	5,6	17	94,4	1			
Gestational age								
< 37 weeks	7	30,4	16	69,6	13,24	2,95	5,95	**0,001**
> 37 weeks	2	2,3	85	97,7	1			
Birth weight in grams								
< 2500	8 0	20,	32	80, 0	14,00	1,8 2	; 10,79	**0,011**
>2500	1	1,4	69	98, 6	1			
Clinical signs of syphilis at birth								
Yes	3	5,0	57	95, 0	2,25	0,2 4	; 20,92	0,476
No	1	2,2	44	97, 8	1			

In the bivariate model involving pregnancy loss with the explanatory variables that showed p<0.20, the following were identified as statistically significant at the 5% level using the stepwise method: marital status (P=0.013), occupation (P=0.005), history of abortion (p<0.001), prenatal care (p<0.001); time with partner in years (p=0.018); gestational age (p=0.001) and birth weight in grams (p=0.011). In other words, the chance of pregnancy loss is: approximately 4 times for those not in a conjugal union; more than 2 times for those with a history of miscarriage; approximately 3 times for those who didn't have prenatal care; almost 8 times for those who didn't have information or didn't have a VDRL test in the 3rd trimester; more than 6 times for those who had inadequate treatment for syphilis; more than 4 times for those who had been with their partner for less than 2 years; more than 13 times for those who had a gestational age of less than 37 weeks and 14 times for those who had a birth weight of less than 2,500 grams (TABLE 4).

Table 4: Bivariate analysis of sociodemographic, gynaecological and obstetric characteristics, current pregnancy, partner and conceptus associated with gestational outcome, candidate variables for the multivariate model. Fortaleza, CE, 2012.

Variables		95% CI		p-value
Marital status				
They don't live together	3,811	,3310	,89	**0,013**
They live together	1			

Occupation				
Unpaid	0,	290, ,	120 68	**0,005**
Paid	1			
Family income in minimum wages				
< 1	0,	150,021 ,06		0,057
> 1	1			
History of abortion				
Yes	5,	212,1312 ,74		**<0,001**
No	1			
Had prenatal care				
No	8,072	,8522	,83	**<0,001**
Yes	1			
VDRL 3rd trimester (n=83)				
Not realised/no information	7,830	,8671	,45	0,068
Realised	1			
Treatment for syphilis				
Inadequate	6,52	0,90	47,08	0,063
Suitable	1			

Table 4: Bivariate analysis of sociodemographic, gynaecological and obstetric characteristics, current pregnancy, partner and conceptus associated with gestational outcome, candidate variables for the multivariate model. Fortaleza, CE, 2012.

Variables		95% CI	p-value
Time with partner in years			
Less than 2	4,46	1,29	**0,018**
2 or more	1		
Gestational age			
< 37 weeks	13,24	2,95	**0,001**
> 37 weeks	1		
Birth weight in grams			
< 2500	14,00	1,82	**0,011**
>2500	1		

Before the final stage of the model, a number of interventions were carried out to remove and add variables:

- It was not possible to estimate the PR for some variables, possibly due to low frequency in some categories;
- It was not possible to estimate the PR for family income and gestational age. In this case, family income was removed as it was of less importance to the situation;
- After removing income, it was not possible to estimate PR for gestational age. So, family income was replaced and gestational age was removed;
- As it was not possible to estimate the PR for the family income variable, it was also removed from the model.

Thus, in the final model involving pregnancy loss with the explanatory variables that showed $p<0.05$ by the stepwise method, the following variables: history of miscarriage ($p=0.008$) PR = 3.11 (adjusted) and 95% CI (1.35; 7.17); prenatal care ($p=0.001$) PR = 5.69 (adjusted) and 95% CI (2.04; 15.83). In other words, the chance of pregnancy loss is: more than 3 times for those with a history of miscarriage and approximately 6 times for those who have not had prenatal care (TABLE 5).

Table 5: Final multivariate model for the outcome gestational loss in women diagnosed with syphilis, Fortaleza-CE, 2012

Variables	Adjusted PR	95% CI	p-value
History of abortion			
Yes	3,11	1,35; 7,17	**0,008**
No	1		
Had prenatal care			
No	5,69	2,04; 15,83	**0,001**
Yes	1		

DISCUSSION

Pregnancy monitoring is essential to ensure the development of the pregnancy period, which in most cases leads to a safe delivery and a healthy newborn (BRASIL, 2012). It was not possible to compare the data on prenatal care due to the scarcity of research on this variable. Ideally, an active search should be made for potential pregnant women with the aim of carrying out 100 per cent of prenatal care and informing them of its importance. It was also observed that the reasons given for not attending prenatal care involved intrinsic issues such as the woman's lack of motivation, as well as a very critical social situation that we all experience at the same time: the explosion of alcohol and other drug users, especially crack cocaine. This fact means that these women are 5.69 times more likely to have a pregnancy loss when compared to pregnant women who have been followed up.

Pregnant women with a gestational age of less than 37 weeks have a 2.95% greater chance of having a negative outcome.

The most frequent place of consultation was the basic health unit (UBS), in line with another study which found that 1,327 pregnant women were consulted (DOMINGUES et al., 2012).

Prenatal care carried out by doctors and nurses is dominant in the study, even though there was a small rate of consultations carried out by just one professional. The need to rotate the service is important, as it takes into account the specificities of the different areas of activity (PEIXOTO et al., 2011).

Low adherence to prenatal care, represented by the low number of appointments made, is a finding also present in other locations, and is one of the main concerns regarding the quality of prenatal care in the country. The number of appointments is at odds with what is recommended by the Ministry of Health, contributing to maternal and child complications (CHAVES et al., 2014).

Early prenatal care is essential for the prevention, detection and treatment of diseases such as syphilis, in order to guarantee the health of the foetus (BRASIL, 2012). However, the study showed that most pregnant women only started their appointments in the second trimester, which is not in line with some studies carried out in other parts of the country in which pregnant women started their follow-up in the first trimester of pregnancy, which is recommended by the Ministry of Health (NONATO; MELO; GUIMARÃES, 2015; MAGALHÃES et al., 2013).

This scenario probably reflects the primary care network in the municipality, with only 35 per cent of the population covered by the Family Health Strategy and 56 per cent by community health agents (FORTALEZA, 2012). This may have a negative impact on the early uptake of pregnant women for prenatal care, providing adequate screening and treatment for syphilis.

The diagnosis of syphilis during prenatal care revealed that the disease was only discovered during prenatal consultations. This data is similar to that found in a study in which 57% of pregnant women were diagnosed with syphilis only during prenatal care (LIMA et al., 2013). However, this is still a low percentage for the rate of discovery of the disease, given that some only find out at the time of delivery, which means that some diseases of concern during pregnancy are being neglected.

The low use of condoms after being diagnosed with the disease often reflects the social culture in which the patient lives. In order to reverse this situation, it would be advisable to develop educational activities to make the partner aware of the need to use this barrier to prevent infection or reinfection.

VDRL serology is the main tool for screening for syphilis and is requested, as a priority, in the first and third trimesters. In the present study there was a prevalence of this case in the quarters mentioned, which is the opposite of a study in which this test was not carried out. The author justifies this data by the fact that blood is not collected at the basic unit, and that the period of consultations is discontinuous, thus weakening the health system (ANVERSA et al., 2012).

Considering that the detection and treatment of syphilis between 24ª and 28ª gestational weeks can be late in preventing complications such as stillbirth or premature births (NASCIMENTO et al., 2012), these findings reinforce the need to invest in the initial prenatal consultation, even in the first trimester, with enough time to implement the protocol for eliminating maternal syphilis and vertical transmission of treponema pallidum, as recommended by the Ministry of Health (BRASIL, 2006).

The partner with syphilis is often considered to be a major facilitator of treatment failure, due to the lack of or inadequate treatment, in addition to the risk of reinfection, if the pregnant woman does not use a condom during the discovery of the disease, as shown in this study (MAGALHÃES et al. 2013; NONATO, MELO, GUIMARÃES, 2015). This study found that not using condoms was more frequent for the outcome of pregnancy loss, which shows how necessary it is to prevent vertical transmission of syphilis.

The short time spent with the partner appears to be an important point because it is associated with the pregnant woman having a 1.29 greater chance of a negative outcome.

The Ministry of Health defines an adequate treatment for syphilis as one in which the pregnant woman has used the correct dose of penicillin for the clinical stage of the disease and has finished her treatment at least 30 days before giving birth, with the partner having been treated concomitantly (BRASIL, 2007b).

In pregnant women, more than half of the treatment, 86 (72.3%), was considered inadequate and 18 (15.1%) resulted in miscarriage or stillbirth. With regard to the outcome of the pregnancy, another study showed convergence, where the outcome was: 67 women, where 15 were pregnant women, 3 had miscarriage as the outcome of the pregnancy, while 52 were puerperal women, two had stillbirths. This shows that gestational syphilis, when not treated properly, can lead to miscarriage and death (MAGALHÃES et al., 2013).

With regard to the mother's age and the outcome, although no statistically significant association was found (p= 0.384), it was observed that 6 (20 per cent) women under the age of 20 had a pregnancy loss, representing the highest percentage among them.

The establishment of colour does not influence the gestational outcome, but a prevalence of brown/black race was found, corroborating a study in which 728 cases were of this race (CALÁS; ANDRADE, 2015). This data may vary according to each region due to the miscegenation of races.

In this study, we found that low schooling predominated among the pregnant women who took part in the research and this is similar to other studies. The author emphasises the value of this sociodemographic information, which shows the social inequality interconnected with the disease (NASCIMENTO, 2012; CALÁS; ANDRADE, 2015).

Marital status was significantly associated ($p=0.013$), showing that women without a stable union may have 1.3 more chances of an unfavourable gestational outcome and, as it was significant in all the stages of building the explanatory model, it was considered important in the final model.

As far as occupation is concerned, the majority of women worked in the home or in informal jobs, and were therefore unpaid. This condition can be understood as a reflection of low schooling, limiting access to the formal labour market. This background had an impact on the outcome ($p=0.005$) showing the negative influence of occupation on pregnancy loss.

When examining the characteristics of the foetus, low birth weight and prematurity predominated. The gestational age of the foetus showed a statistically significant association ($p=0.011$) with the outcome. This finding is in line with the study by Nascimento et al. (2012), who carried out a study in a hospital on complicated pregnancies affected by maternal syphilis, and found that the majority of pregnancies, 32 (66.7%), had a preterm foetal death outcome.

A history of miscarriage plays a negative role in the outcome ($p=0.008$), which goes against the data found in a study showing a low rate of miscarriages among pregnant women (LINS, 2014).

CONCLUSION

The study revealed a very complex situation that includes failures in the health service, late testing for syphilis and inadequate treatment. In addition to the fact that the prenatal care routine is not being carried out properly, the persistence of the obstacle of not treating the partner and the underreporting of cases signalled missed opportunities to control the disease.

The significant associations found throughout the study showed an interaction between social, biological and health care factors in maintaining vertical transmission of syphilis as a public health problem, determined by the following variables: marital status, occupation, history of abortion, prenatal care, time with partner in years, gestational age, birth weight in grams.

It was found that women who had a history of miscarriage and had not had prenatal care had a higher risk of having a pregnancy loss.

It is necessary to make progress in the organisation of health services, to increase the early recruitment of pregnant women, to increase adherence to prenatal care, to make the routine of tests recommended by the Ministry of Health feasible and to guarantee the appropriate and timely treatment of pregnant women and their partners when they test positive for syphilis.It is important to delve deeper into comparative studies to better assess this important component of perinatal morbidity and mortality in the country. There is also a need for actions in care, from the perspective of comprehensive health care, with a view to overcoming the problems identified, making it possible to reverse the unfavourable situation of vertical transmission of syphilis.

REFERENCES

ALMEIDA, F.C.M. **Vertical transmission of syphilis: an analysis of the factors involved in morbidity and mortality**, 2012. 74f. Dissertation (Master's in Public Health) - Health Science Centre, State University of Ceará, 2012.

ANVERSA, E.T.R.; et al. Quality of the prenatal care process: basic health units and Family Health Strategy units in a municipality in southern Brazil. **Cadernos de Saúde Pública,** v.28, n.4, p.789-800, 2012.

BARROS, A.; HIRAKATA, V.N. Alternatives for logistic regressio n in cross- sectional studies: an empirical comparison of models that directly estimate the prevalence ratio. **Bmc Medical Research Methodology,** v.21, n.3, p.1-13, 2003.

BRAZIL. Ministry of Health. Low-risk prenatal care. Brasília: Ministry of Health, 2012 (Primary Care Notebooks, n. 32).

BRAZIL. Ministry of Health. Child health: growth and development. Brasília: Ministry of Health, 2012 (Primary Care Notebooks, n. 33).

BRAZIL. Ministry of Health. Health Surveillance Secretariat. **Protocol for the prevention of vertical transmission of HIV and syphilis** - pocket manual. Brasília, 2007. 190 p.

BRAZIL. Ministry of Health. Health Surveillance Secretariat. National STD/AIDS Programme. **Guidelines for the control of congenital syphilis:** pocket manual. 2. ed. Brasília, 2006. 72 p. (Manual Series 24).

CALÁS, J.E.S.; ANDRADE, C.L.T. **Gestational syphilis in selected municipalities of Metropolitan Region I of the State of Rio de Janeiro, 2011 to 2013.** 2015. 77 f. Dissertation (Master's Degree) - Public Health Course, Sergio Arouca National School of Public Health, Rio de Janeiro.

CAMPOS, A.L.A.; et al. Syphilis in parturients: aspects related to the sexual partner. **Revista Brasileira de Ginecologia e Obstetrícia**, v.34, n.9, p.397-402, 2012.

CARVALHO, I.S.; BRITO, R.S. Congenital syphilis in Rio Grande do Norte: a descriptive study of the period 2007-2010. **Epidemiologia e Serviços de Saúde**, v.23, n.2, p.287-294, 2014.

CEARÁ. GOVERNMENT OF THE STATE OF CEARÁ. **Epidemiological Report:** Congenital Syphilis. Fortaleza, 2013. 12 p.

COSTA, C.C.; et al. Congenital syphilis in Ceará: epidemiological analysis of a decade. **Revista da Escola de Enfermagem da USP**, v.47, n.1, p.152- 159, 2013.

CHAVES, J.; et al. Congenital syphilis: analysis of a hospital in the interior of the state of RS. **Revista da Amrigs**, v.3, n.58, p.187-192, 2014.

COUTINHO, L.M.S.; SCARZUFCA, M.; MENENZES, P.R. Methods for estimating prevalence ratios in cross-sectional studies. **Revista de Saúde Pública,** v.42, n.6, p.992-998, 2008.

DOMINGUES, R.M.S.M.; et al. Evaluation of the adequacy of prenatal care in the SUS network of the Municipality of Rio de Janeiro, Brazil. **Cadernos de Saúde Pública,** v.28, n.3, p.425-437, 2012.

DOMINGUES, R.M.S.M.; et al. Prevalence of syphilis during pregnancy and prenatal testing: A study born in Brazil. **Revista de Saúde Pública**, v.48, n.5, p.766-774, 2014.

FORTALEZA. Municipal Health Department. **Coverage of the Family Health Programme**. Fortaleza, 2012.

FORTALEZA. Municipal Health Department. **Fortaleza Health Bulletin**, v.13, n.3, 2009.

HOSMER, D.W.; LEMESHOW, S. **Applied logistic regression**. New York: Wiley, 1989.

LIMA, M.G.; et al. Incidence and risk factors for congenital syphilis in Belo Horizonte, Minas Gerais, 2001-2008. **Ciência & Saúde Coletiva**, v.2, n.18, p.499-506, 2013.

LINS, C.D.M. **Epidemiology of gestational and congenital syphilis in the far northern Amazon.** 2014. 72f. Dissertation (Master's) - Professional Master's Programme, Federal University of Roraima, Boa Vista.

MAGALHÃES, D.M.S.; et al. Maternal and congenital syphilis: still a challenge. **Cadernos de Saúde Pública**, v.6, n.29, p.1109-1120, 2013.

NASCIMENTO, M.I.; et al. Pregnancies complicated by maternal syphilis and foetal death. **Revista Brasileira de Ginecologia e Obstetrícia**, v.34, n.2, p.56-62, 2012.

NONATO, S.M.; MELO, A.P.S.; GUIMARÃES, M.D.C. Syphilis during pregnancy and factors associated with congenital syphilis in Belo Horizonte-MG, 2010-2013. **Epidemiologia em Serviços de Saúde**, Brasília, v.4, n.24, p.681-694, 2015.

PEIXOTO, C.R.; et al. Prenatal care in primary care: the starting point for reorganising obstetric care. **Revista de Enfermagem**, Rio de Janeiro, v.19, n.2, p.286-291, 2011.

SILVA, A.R.; CASTRO, A.R. **Epidemiological profile of pregnant women diagnosed with syphilis in Brazil (2005 to 2012), with evidence in the Federal District. 2013.** 17f. TCC (Graduation) - Biomedicine Course, Faculdades Integradas Icesp/Promove de BrasÍlia.

VICTORA, C.G.; et al. Longitudinal study of the mother and child population in the urban region of Southern Brazil, 1993: methodological aspects and preliminary results. **Revista de Saúde Pública,** v. 30, n. 1, p.34-35, nov. 1996.

WORLD HEALTH ORGANISATION. Investment case for eliminating mother-to- child transmission of syphilis: promoting better maternal and child health and stronger health systems. Geneva; 2012.

CHAPTER 5

CONGENITAL MALFORMATION: characteristics of mothers and live births

Selma Antunes Nunes Diniz

Juliana Alencar Moreira Borges

Geziel dos Santos Sousa

Francisco José Maia Pinto

Débora Sâmara Guimarães Dantas

Rafaella Maria Monteiro Sampaio

Francisco Regis da Silva

INTRODUCTION

In the international context, Brazil has adopted the targets of the Millennium Development Goals, one of which is to reduce child mortality. In Millennium Development Goal 4, the target was to reduce mortality among children under five by two thirds between 1990 and 2015. From 1990, the base year for comparing progress on the Millennium Development Goals (MDGs), until 2008, the average national reduction was 58 per cent, with differences between regions (BRASIL, 2011a).

Also according to Brasil (2011a), infant mortality, an indicator of the population's living conditions and health, although it has been falling progressively in Brazil, is still below the target. Special efforts on the part of the entire population, especially health services and professionals, are important in order to accelerate its reduction and achieve more virtuous rates for the Brazilian population.

In Ceará there is also a downward trend in the Infant Mortality Rate (IMR), from 32 deaths per 1,000 live births (LB) in 1997 to 13.1 in 2010. Neonatal infant mortality has been falling, but more slowly, exceeding the post-neonatal IMR. In 2010, 1,691 deaths of children under one year of age were reported, 71.4 per cent (1,691) neonatal. In the same year, 128,831 children were born (CEARÁ, 2012).

In the municipality of Fortaleza, the IMR is also on a downward trend. Between 1981 and 2013, the Infant Mortality Rate fell from 101.5 deaths per thousand live births in 1981 to 11.7 in 2013. This decrease is due to factors associated with improved living conditions, public interventions in the areas of health and education, and even improvements in infrastructure and basic sanitation, among other factors (FORTALEZA, 2014).

The fall in infant mortality due to infectious, parasitic and respiratory diseases revealed an increase in the relative share of Congenital Malformations (CM) in infant deaths, while other causes of death were controlled, they took on a proportionally greater role (GEREMIAS; ALMEIDA; FLORES, 2009).

CBMs or congenital defects are all functional or structural anomalies of foetal development, resulting from factors originating before birth, from genetic, environmental or unknown causes, even if the defect is not visible in the newborn (NB) or becomes evident later (RAMOS; CORRADINI; NEME, 1974).

Around 3% of live births in the world and in Brazil have some kind of malformation detected at birth, either totally or partially due to genetic factors (HOROVITZ; LLERENA; MATTOS, 2005; GUERRA et al., 2008). The general incidence of CBM in South America is 5%, similar to other regions of the world (GOMES; COSTA, 2012).

In the municipality of Fortaleza-Ceará, according to data from the Information Department of the Unified Health System (DATASUS), CBMs are in 2nd place among the other causes of death in children under one year old (FORTALEZA, 2013).

In view of the above, the aim of this study was to describe the characteristics of mothers and live births with congenital malformations in the municipality of Fortaleza-CE between 2001 and 2010.

METHODS

This was a case-control study, characterised by the fact that it is an observational study that begins by selecting a group of people with a specific disease or condition (cases) and another group of people not affected by that disease or condition (controls). The proportion of people exposed to a risk factor is measured in both groups and compared (MEDRONHO et al., 2009).

The study took place in the municipality of Fortaleza, at the Municipal Health Department (SMS), by consulting the Live Birth Information System (SINASC) and the Mortality Information System (SIM), from 01/01/2001 to 31/12/2010.

The study population consisted of all live births with a Certificate of Live Birth (CLB), totalling 389,904, and all deaths in children under one year old (6,811) recorded on Death Certificates (DC) in the municipality of Fortaleza (SMS - TABNET, Fortaleza).

The basis for calculating the sample comprised all DNV's (2,231 births) with a mention of congenital malformation, and all deaths (1,079 with a CBM (PART I of the DC), plus 93 deaths with a mention of CBM (PART II of the DC), totalling 1,172 deaths (SMS - TABNET, Fortaleza).

Excluded from the sample were births with CBM that progressed to infant death in 2001 and were born in 2000, as well as the DCs of children of mothers living outside Fortaleza. The final sample totalled 2,052, with 513 cases and 1,539 controls, corresponding to three times the number of cases.

The cases and controls in this study were defined using the SINASC and SIM information systems, according to the following flowchart:

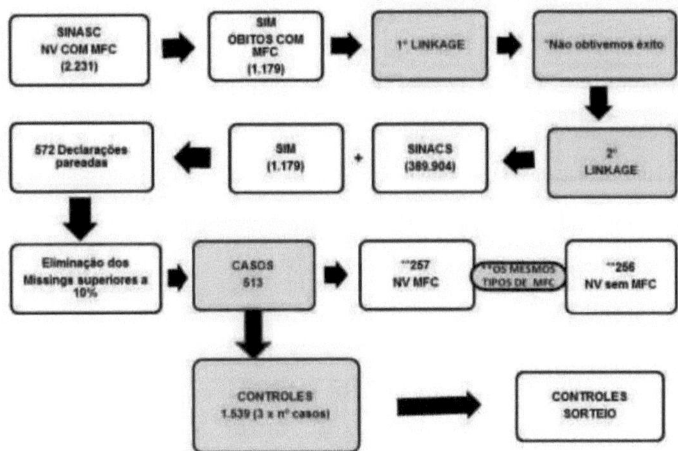

Figure 1: Cases and controls defined from SINASC and SIM

The variables used were classified as outcome and explanatory. The outcome was represented by infant death with congenital malformation (occurring in the neonatal and post-neonatal period), and the explanatory variables were configured in the three hierarchical blocks, according to the conceptual model.

In this research, the data was distributed in three blocks:

a) Block 1 - distal level: characteristics of the mother's socioeconomic and demographic profile

These variables are considered to be the most distant in the model, given that most of the time their effects on infant death are no longer statistically significant in the presence of intermediate and proximal level variables (LIMA; CARVALHO; VASCONCELOS, 2008).

- **Maternal age (<20 and >20 years old);**
- **Years of study (<4 and £4 years);**
- Marital status (living together, not living together);

I HDI (low/medium - 0 to 0.732; high - >0.733 and <1).

b) Block 2 - intermediate level: maternal characteristics and characteristics relating to prenatal care and childbirth

These variables make up the intermediate level because they show effects whose magnitude is reduced when the proximal variables are included (LIMA; CARVALHO; VASCONCELOS, 2008).

- Gestational age (<37, > 37 weeks);

8 Type of pregnancy (single, multiple);

9 N° of births (primiparous and multiparous);

- **No. of miscarriages (none, >1);**
- N° of **antenatal** consultations **(<7, >7);**

8 Type of birth (vaginal caesarean).

c) Block 3 - proximal: newborn health conditions and neonatal care

The variables at the proximal level, the biological factors of the NB, stand out as the main predictors of infant death (LIMA; CARVALHO; VASCONCELOS, 2008).

- **Age at death (<7, >7 days);**
- **Birth weight (<2500, >2500 grams);**
- **Apgar score at 10 minutes (<7, >7);**
- **Apgar score at 50 minutes (<7, >7);**

8 Type of congenital malformation;

s Sex (male and female).

Microsoft Office Excel version 7.0 was used to tabulate the data, and the data was double-entered in order to detect possible inconsistencies. The STATA programme, version 11.0, and the ***TabNet - Web*** programme from the Fortaleza-CE Municipal Health Department were used to process the general data.

The general data was analysed descriptively using frequencies (absolute and relative) and parametric measures (mean and standard deviation).

Inferential analysis was carried out to verify the association between risk factors for infant mortality due to congenital malformations in the neonatal and post-neonatal periods, using the chi-square test, Maximum Likelihood, at a significance level of 5%, for the qualitative variables distributed in the three hierarchical blocks.

The strength of association between the variables was estimated using bivariate analysis involving the Odds Ratio.

To control for possible confounding factors in the associations obtained from the bivariate analysis, the multiple logistic regression technique was used, adopting the descriptive value $p<0.20$ as a way of selecting the variables to enter the model and $p<0.05$ as a way of the variable remaining in the model.

Finally, a hierarchical multiple regression model was built for the factors in each block in order to highlight the best adjusted infant mortality at a 5% significance level.

This study is an excerpt from Diniz's dissertation (2014) and followed the recommendations of **Resolution N⁰ 466 of 2012, which regulates "research involving human beings" of the National Health Council and provides guidance** on the procedures to be used when collecting information (BRASIL, 2012).

RESULTS

In Fortaleza, the IMR has been on a steady downward trend, with a reduction from 17.0 deaths per 1,000 live births in 2001 to 12.1/1,000 live births in 2010, which implies a decrease of 28.8% over the period. With regard to Infant Mortality Rates due to Congenital Malformations (IMR), small changes in the increase were noticeable from 2004 onwards, with a small reduction in 2010 (Graph 1).

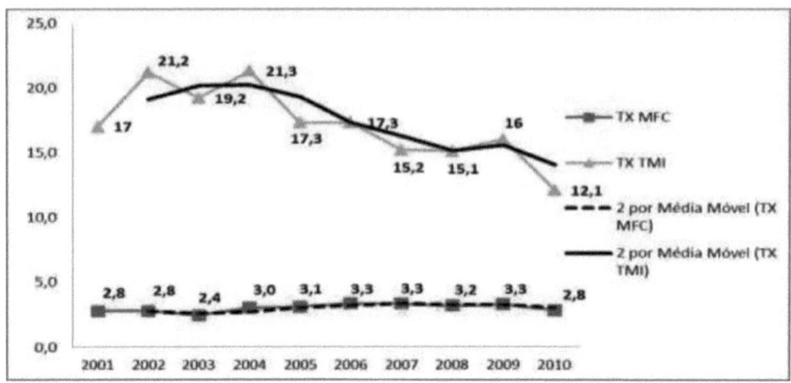

Graph 1: Distribution of the infant mortality rate per thousand live births and the infant mortality rate due to congenital malformations in Fortaleza-CE, BR, between 2001 and 2010.

TX TMI: Infant Mortality Rate.
TX MFC: Infant Mortality Rate due to Congenital Malformation. Source: Tabnet/SMS/Fortaleza - SINASC/SIM.

In the sample surveyed, all live births had congenital malformations, and this was checked by filling in field 34 (presence of anomaly, yes or no).

When it came to deaths with CBM, it was noted that although all of them had died, not all of them had field 34 filled in on their respective DN. Through linkage, it was possible to identify these declarations and see how fragile it is to fill in these official documents.

In the group of cases, SINASC reported 257 (50.09%) cases of CBM and SIM reported 246 (49.90%), meaning that SIM proved to be a very important information system for retrieving CBM data in the study.

The results of this study were drawn, following the hierarchical model for the study of infant death with CBM (outcome), from the distal, intermediate and proximal levels. Table 1 contains the distal level variables relating to the outcome of infant death with CBM, the mother's socioeconomic and demographic characteristics.

Table 1: Unadjusted distal risk factors for infant mortality with congenital malformation, according to mothers' socioeconomic and demographic characteristics, Fortaleza, CE, BR, 2001 to 2010.

VARIABLES	CASE		CONTROL		OR no adjusted	95% CI	P
	n (=513)	%	n (=1.539)	%			
Maternal age							

>20 years	99	19,30	330	21,44	1,0		
< 20 years	414	80,70	1.209	78,56	0,87	0,68; 1,12	0,30
Years of study							
>4 years	289	58,09	929	60,10	1,0		
<4 years	215	41,91	614	39,90	1,08	0,88; 1,33	0,42
Marital status							
Live together	123	23,98	403	26,19	1,0		
Not living together	390	76,02	1.136	73,81	1,12	0,89; 1,41	0,32
HDI							
Medium/High	295	57,50	-	-			
Bass	218	42,50	-	-			

95% CI: 95% confidence interval; OR: odds ratio; P-value < 0.05. Source: SINASC/SIM.

The inferential analysis revealed that the mean maternal age was 26 ± 7.14 years, with a minimum age of 12 and a maximum of 47. Most of the mothers were under 20 years old, both in the cases [414 (80.70%)] and in the controls [1209 (78.56%) (OR=0.87; CI 0.68; 1.12)].

The majority of mothers had four or more years of schooling, both in cases [289 (58.09%)] and controls [929 (60.10%)], with (OR=1.08; CI 0.88; 1.33), and were not living with a partner [390 (76.02%)] in cases and [1136 (73.81%)] in controls, with (OR=1.12; CI 0.89; 1.41). As for the HDI, [295 (57.50%)] of the cases had values between medium and high.

With regard to the intermediate level, which refers to mothers' characteristics about pregnancy and childbirth, the following variables were analysed: gestational age, type of pregnancy, number of births, number of abortions, prenatal consultations, type of childbirth and number of prenatal consultations. Table 2 shows the intermediate level of the hierarchical model.

More than half of the time, the following were observed: gestational age > 37 weeks for cases [313 (61.01%)] and controls [1172 (76.15%)] (OR= 2.04; CI 1.64; 2.53); type of single pregnancy in cases and controls with [490 (95.52%)] and [1484 (96.43%)] (OR=1.26; CI 0.77; 2.08); number of births (multiparous) among cases [361 (70.37%)] and controls [1043 (67.77%)] (OR=0.88; CI 0.71; 1.10); the number of women who did not have an abortion, in cases [294 (57.31%)] and controls [933 (60.62%)] (OR=1.14; CI 0.93; 1.40); caesarean delivery in cases [279 (54.39%)] and controls [858(55.57%)]

(OR=0.94; CI 0.77; 1.15); number of antenatal care visits <7 in cases [365 (71.15%)] and controls [1072 (69.66%)] (OR=0.95; CI 0.76; 1.18); as for the health establishments where the birth took place, [453(88.3%)] were in public/accredited hospitals.

Table 2: Unadjusted intermediate risk factors for infant mortality with congenital malformation, according to maternal characteristics, Fortaleza, CE, BR, 2001 to 2010.

VARIABLES	CASE		CONTROL		Unadjusted OR	95% CI	P
	n (=513)	%	n (=1536)	%			
Gestational age (weeks)							
>37	31361	,01	1.17276	,15	1,0		
< 37	38,99	200	36723	,85	2,04	1,64; 2,53	**<0,001**
Type of pregnancy							
Unique	49095	,52	1.48496	,43	1,0		
Multiple	48	234,	553	,57	1,26	0,77; 2,08	0,35
Number of births							
Primipara	152	29,63	496	32,23	1,0		
Multiparous	361	70,37	1.043	67,77	0,88	0,71; 1,10	0,27
Number of miscarriages							
None	294	57,31	933	60,62	1,0		
>1	219	42,69	606	39,38	1,14	0,93; 1,40	0,18
Type of labour							
Vaginal	234	45,51	681	44,25	1,0		
Cesario	279	54,39	858	55,57	0,94	0,77; 1,15	0,59
No. of PN consultations							
>7	8	14 28,8	467	30,34	1,0		
< 7	5	36 71,1	2 1.07	69,66	5 0,9	0,76; 1,18	0,65
Establishments Health			-	-	-	-	-
Private	60	11,70					
Public/convened	353	88,30					

95% CI: 95% confidence interval; OR: odds ratio. P-value < 0.05 Source: SINASC/SIM.

The univariate analysis of block 2 showed that only gestational age (less than 37 weeks) was associated with the outcome, with a value of p<0.001, meeting the criterion of p<0.20 to take part in the next stage of the study.

The block of variables at the proximal level involved the characteristics of the newborns, such as age at death, birth weight, Apgar score at the first and fifth minute and gender.

More than half of the deaths studied occurred: [229 (50.89%)] in the early neonatal period (0 to 6 days), i.e. in the first week of life; with birth weight £ 2500g, in cases [279 (54.39%)] and controls [1162 (75.50%)] (OR=2.58; CI 2.08; 3.19); APGAR index at 1 minute < 7 in cases was [262 (51.07%)] (OR 2.58; CI 3.03; 4.71), while in controls > 7 it was [1.206 (78.36%), (OR=28.24; CI 15.00; 53.18); at the 5th minute, the index > 7 in cases and controls was [374 (72.90%) and 1,423 (92.46%), respectively, with (OR= 4.55; CI 3.44; 6.03) and males in cases [238 (50.28%)] and controls [844 (50.84%)]. The average weight of the NBs was 2,126g, with a standard deviation of 1,027g, the minimum weight being 620g and the maximum 3,900g (Table 3).

Table 3: Characteristics of newborn health conditions and neonatal care, Fortaleza, CE, BR, 2001 to 2010.

VARIABLES	CASE		CONTROL		OR no adjusted	95% CI	P
	n=(513*)	%	n=(1539)	%			
Age at death (days)							
Early neonatal	229	50,89	-	-	-	-	-
Late Neonatal	13	2,89	-	-	-	-	-
Post-neonatal	208	46,22	-	-	-	-	-
Birth weight (g)							
>2500	279	54,39	1.162	75,50	1,0		
< 2500	234	45,61	377	24,50	2,58	2,08; 3,19	**<0,001**
APGAR 1st minute							
>7	251	48,93	1.206	78,36	1,0		
< 7	262	51,07	333	21,64	3,78	3,03; 4,71	**<0,001**
APGAR 5th minute							
>7	374	72,90	1.423	92,46	1,0		
< 7	139	27,1	116	7,54	4,55	3,44; 6,03	**<0,001**

		0					
Sex							
Male	238	50,28	844	54,84	-	-	-
Female	242	41,17	662	43,01	-	-	-

95% CI: 95% confidence interval; OR: Odds Ratio. P-value < 0.05
* Note: In the age at death variable, the sample presented did not correspond to the sample size established for the survey, due to the fact that the age at death was not filled in on the DC. Source: SINASC/SIM.

In block 3, the variables birth weight, APGAR at 1 minute and APGAR at 5 minutes were associated with the outcome, with a value of p<0.001, meeting the criterion of p<0.20 to take part in the next stage of the study.

DISCUSSION

Information on mortality is relevant for epidemiological and demographic studies of a country's population, as well as for the planning and management of health policies and actions, and it is essential that it is reliable and accessible (DINIZ, 2014).

The Births (SINASC) and Mortality (SIM) Information Systems record and process data on vital statistics. In addition to the numbers of live births and deaths, which allow for the direct calculation of important health indicators, such as infant mortality, SINASC and SIM provide other essential information, such as: characteristics of the mother's socioeconomic and demographic profile, characteristics relating to prenatal care and childbirth, and health conditions of the newborn and neonatal care, respectively (DRUMOND; MACHADO; FRANÇA, 2007).

This work revealed that the probabilistic linkage between the SIM and SINASC databases is viable, feasible and fruitful, especially when it comes to observing certain situations, including the failure to fill in field 34 of the DN (yes and no) (DINIZ, 2014).

Also according to Diniz (2014), when the linkage showed that almost half of the 513 cases in the study (49.91 per cent) had not filled in field 34, it was possible to retrieve information and, therefore, get a closer estimate of the prevalence of CBM in live births.

As for the reduction in IMR shown in this study, it was observed that there was a considerable decline in the decade studied. According to the Ministry of Health, the infant mortality rate (under one year of age) in Brazil has been falling progressively since 1990, from 47.1 deaths for every thousand babies born alive to 19.3 deaths in 2007, a reduction of 59.7 per cent over this period (BRASIL, 2011b).

Therefore, if the municipality of Fortaleza continues to reduce these figures, or even maintains them, it will achieve the fourth target of the Millennium Development Goals (MDGs), which is to reduce child mortality to 15.7/1000 LB by 2015 (UNICEF, 2007).

On the other hand, it was observed that the infant mortality rate due to congenital malformations has been showing an increase since 2004, **continuing until 2010. In the study "Infant mortality due to congenital malformations** in Brazil, **1996-2008", Siedersberger Neto et al.** (2012) emphasise that the current trend in various regions of the world is evidenced by the reduction in the infant mortality rate, in contrast to the proportional increase in infant deaths due to congenital malformations.

The infant deaths with congenital malformations presented in this study show that the neonatal component provides the highest percentage of infant mortality, which corroborates the results found in other **studies. Gomes and Costa (2012) in their study on "Infant mortality and** congenital malformations in the Municipality of Pelotas, State of Rio Grande do Sul, Brazil: ecological study in the period **1996-2008" it was observed** that the main reasons for deaths in Pelotas-RS occurred in the perinatal period and, thus, according to the proportional distribution of infant deaths investigated in the place under study, it was found that the late neonatal component made up the most prevalent infant death component, corresponding to 49.2 per cent of deaths, followed by the early neonatal (35.6 per cent) and post neonatal (15.3 per cent) components. Thus, the early neonatal period was the largest component of the infant mortality rate found.

In Brazil, the reduction in infant mortality has fundamentally occurred in the post-neonatal component, due to various actions, including immunoprevention and encouraging breastfeeding. Currently, the challenge for health policies is to reduce neonatal mortality, especially the early neonatal component, which ensures the survival of newborns during this critical period for their health (BORGES, 2012).

In this study, the risk factors for neonatal mortality were described and categorised according to the hierarchical model already described.

In this model, risk factors are classified into three blocks - block 1 - distal level: characteristics of the mother's socioeconomic and demographic profile; block 2 - intermediate level: maternal characteristics (reproductive history, maternal morbidity and behaviour, characteristics relating to prenatal care and childbirth) and block 3 - proximal level: health conditions of the newborn and neonatal care.

Applying the model to this study, with regard to the maternal age variable, cases and controls showed a predominance of teenage pregnancies, i.e. in children under 20 years of age. It was found that maternal age was a decisive parameter for the incidence of CBM, as the incidence of CBM occurred in both cases and controls (DINIZ, 2014).

Brazilian authors have found a relationship between maternal age and congenital malformation in adolescent mothers and have concluded that the chances of an adolescent with multiple pregnancies having a child with a malformation is 6.14 times higher when compared to adolescents with a single pregnancy (BRITO et al., 2010).

With regard to the maternal schooling variable, it was found that the majority of mothers, in both cases and controls, had studied for four years or more. Similar results were highlighted by Jobim and Aerts (2008) in their study on preventable infant mortality and associated factors in Porto Alegre, where they studied 1,139 "deaths of children for whom a Death Certificate (DC) was issued"; as a result, they realised that the majority of mothers, 514 (45.1%), had between four and seven years of schooling.

This demonstrates the improvement in socio-economic conditions reflected in various aspects of society; the increase in maternal schooling gives women a different view of their health and that of their families. Education is fundamental for people to take responsibility for their health/disease process. Therefore, mothers with more years of schooling showed greater protection against neonatal death.

The mothers' marital status is also described in this block. Most of them are not living with their partner.

When observing the HDI of deaths from CBM by neighbourhood, it was found that (57.50%) are in the medium/high range of human development, when the HDI was compared by the set of neighbourhoods of the Regional Offices of Fortaleza, there was an inversion in the association, i.e. the higher the HDI, the lower the number of deaths from CBM (DINIZ, 2014).

In this study, gestational age greater than or equal to 37 weeks was a preponderant factor between cases and controls. Children born at less than 37 weeks of gestation were at twice the risk of dying from congenital malformations.

The single pregnancy type was dominant in both cases and controls, appearing as a protective factor against neonatal death. Multiple gestation resulted in a 1.26 times greater risk of death from CBM.

As for the number of miscarriages, mothers who had no miscarriages predominated, but among mothers who had at least one miscarriage, the prevalence was in the control group.

Preventing disabilities is one of the prenatal care guidelines. However, poor care for pregnant women has been responsible for 16.8 per cent of the births of children with a certain disability, followed by genetic problems, with 16.6 per cent (BRITO et al., 2010).

In this study, the majority of mothers, among cases and controls, had fewer than seven antenatal visits, contrary to the recommendations of the Ministry of Health, which considers the minimum number of visits to be adequate for low-risk antenatal care. The fact that the number of prenatal consultations was less than seven led to a higher number of children with CBMs resulting from the nervous system, with anencephaly being the most prevalent type. This neural tube disorder can be prevented with the use of folic acid during prenatal care (DINIZ, 2014).

The deaths of NBs with CBM (88.3%) occurred in public establishments. In the study by Ribeiro **et al.** (2009), in Recife (PE), on **"Risk factors for** neonatal **mortality** in children with low **birth** weight**", birth in a SUS hospital was shown to be** a risk factor for neonatal mortality in children with low birth weight.

A birth weight of less than 2,500g resulted in a 2.6 greater risk of dying from CFM. Corroborating this result, Mombelli **et al.** (2012), in their study **"Risk factors for infant mortality in municipalities in the state of Paraná, from 1997 to 2008", reported that low birth weight babies were 4.9 times more** likely to die than those weighing 2500g or more.

The APGAR variables at the 1st and 5th minutes were also significant, after statistical adjustment. These results are corroborated in the study by Geib **et al.** (2010), in which live births with an Apgar score of less than seven in the fifth minute of life had an 8.7 times greater risk of death than those with scores greater than seven.

The results of this study reveal a higher mortality rate among male newborns. Female gender emerged as a protective factor for neonatal mortality, corroborating the data available in the literature.

CONCLUSION

The study found that the infant mortality rate showed a progressive drop, while the infant mortality rate due to congenital malformations remained constant when compared with mortality in children under one year old and increased, with a small variation, when assessed in isolation. More than half of the deaths from congenital malformations occurred in the neonatal component, with a greater preponderance in the early neonatal period.

The use of secondary data proved to be a limiting factor in this research, when information on certain variables was found to be missing, as well as duplicates in the SIM and SINASC databases. However, this did not invalidate the analysis and its results.

The study offers promising prospects for further research of this kind, which will improve both the quality of information and the implementation of policies aimed at reducing infant mortality.

REFERENCES

BORGES JAM. Study of gestational drug addiction and neonatal death. 2012. Dissertation (Master's) - State University of Ceará, Fortaleza, 2012.

BRAZIL. National Health Council. Resolution no. 466, of 12 December 2012. Brasília, 2012.

BRAZIL. Ministry of Health. Health Care Secretariat. Department of Programme and Strategic Actions. **Newborn health care**: a guide for health professionals. Brasília: Ministry of Health, 2011a.

BRAZIL. Ministry of Health. **An analysis of the health situation and evidence of the impact of health surveillance actions**. Infant mortality in Brazil: trends, components and causes of death from 2000 to 2010. Brasília, 2011b. p.117-134.

BRITO VRdeS; et al. Congenital malformations and maternal risk factors in Campina Grande-Paraíba. **Revista Rene**, Fortaleza, v.11, n.2, p.1-212, 2010.

CEARÁ. Ceará State Health Department. **State Health Plan 2012-2015**. Fortaleza, 2012.

DINIZ SAN. **Infant mortality and association with congenital malformation**: a decade-long analysis. 2014. 78f. Dissertation (Master's in Collective Health) - State University of Ceará, Fortaleza, 2014.

DRUMOND EF; MACHADO CJ; FRANÇA E. Early neonatal deaths: analysis of multiple causes of death using the Grade of Membership method. **Cadernos de Saúde Pública**, Rio de Janeiro, v.23, n.1, p.157-166, 2007.

FORTALEZA. Municipal Health Department. **Tab net information**. Available at: <http://www.saudefortaleza.ce.gov.br.

FORTALEZA. Municipal Health Department. **Fortaleza Municipal Health Plan 2014-2017**. Fortaleza, 2014.

UNITED NATIONS CHILDREN'S FUND-UNICEF. **State of the World's**

Children 2008: child survival. Brasilia, 2007.

GEIB LTC; FRÉU CM; BRANDÃO M; NUNES ML. Social and biological determinants of infant mortality in a population-based cohort in Passo Fundo, Rio Grande do Sul. **Ciência & Saúde Coletiva**, Rio de Janeiro, v.15, p.363-370, 2010.

GEREMIAS AL; ALMEIDA MF; FLORES LPO. Evaluation of live birth certificates as a source of information on birth defects. **Revista Brasileira de Epidemiologia**, v.12, n.1, p.60-68, 2009.

GOMES MRR; COSTA JSDda. Infant mortality and congenital malformations in the municipality of Pelotas, state of Rio Grande do Sul, Brazil: an ecological study from 1996-2008. **Epidemiologia e Serviços de Saúde**, Brasília, v.21, n.1, p.119-128, 2012.

GUERRA FAR; LLERENA JRJC; GAMA SGN; CUNHA CB; THEME FILHA MM. Birth defects in the municipality of Rio de Janeiro, Brazil: an evaluation through SINASC: 2000-2004. **Cadernos de Saúde Pública**, Rio de Janeiro, v.24, p.140-149, 2008.

HOROVITZ DDG; LLERENA JRJC; MATTOS RA. Attention to birth defects in Brazil: current panorama. **Cadernos de Saúde Pública**, Rio de Janeiro, v.21, n. 4, p.1055-1064, 2005.

JOBIM R; AERTS D. Preventable Infant Mortality and Associated Factors. **Cadernos de Saúde Pública**, Rio de Janeiro, v.24, p.179-189, jan, 2008.

LIMA S; CARVALHO ML; VASCONCELOS AGG. Proposal for a hierarchical model applied to the investigation of risk factors for neonatal infant death. **Cadernos de Saúde Pública**, Rio de Janeiro, v.24, p.1910-1916, aug, 2008.

MEDRONHO RA; BLOCH KV. (Editor-in-Chief) (Editor). **Epidemiology**. 2. ed. São Paulo, SP: Atheneu, 2009. 493p.

MOMBELLI MA; et al. Risk factors for infant mortality in municipalities in the state of Paraná, from 1997 to 2008. **Revista Paulista de Pediatria**, São Paulo, v.30, n.2, p.187-194, 2012.

RAMOS JLA; CORRADINI HB; NEME B. Malformations. In: ALCÂNTARA P; MARCONDES E; et al. **Basic Paediatrics**. São Paulo: Sarvier, 1974. v.2, p. 1614-1616.

RIBEIRO AM; et al. Risk factors for neonatal mortality in low birth weight infants. **Revista de Saúde Pública**, São Paulo, v.43, n.2, p.246-255, 2009.

SIEDERSBERGER NETO P; ZHANG L; NICOLETTI D; BARTH FM. Infant mortality due to congenital malformations in Brazil, 1996-2008. **Revista da AMRIGS**, Porto Alegre, v.56, n.2, p.129-132, 2012.

CHAPTER 6

EPIDEMIOLOGICAL PROFILE OF INFANT MORTALITY IN FORTALEZA - CEARÁ

Lídia Samara de Castro Sanders
Francisco José Maia Pinto
Rafaella Maria Monteiro Sampaio
Radmila Alves Alencar Viana
Katherine Jeronimo Lima
Ana Maria Peixoto Cabral Maia

INTRODUCTION

The infant mortality rate (IMR) is a classic indicator of a population's level of health, social and economic development. Monitoring the evolution of this rate is essential for drawing up public policies aimed at promoting children's health. Over the years, Brazil has shown a downward trend, reducing infant deaths by 39 per cent between 2000 and 2010. This scenario was common to all Brazilian regions, especially the Northeast, which fell by 48 per cent in the same period (BRASIL, 2012).

The development of socio-economic policies and advances in the care provided by health services have a direct impact on IMR and its determining factors (NASCIMENTO et al., 2012).

IMR can also be assessed according to its components, such as early and late neonatal and post-neonatal, as the causes of infant mortality vary according to the age of the child. The neonatal component (up to 27 days after birth) is a very vulnerable period in the baby's life due to the influence of biological, social, cultural and environmental risk factors. It is mainly related to the care provided to pregnant women during prenatal care, childbirth and newborn care. The main underlying causes of neonatal mortality are congenital anomalies, perinatal conditions and complications during pregnancy, such as hypertension and gestational diabetes, and during labour, such as intrauterine anoxia. The post-neonatal component is related to socio-economic conditions and childcare. The main underlying causes of death in this age group are respiratory problems, gastroenteritis and malnutrition (BRASIL, 2011; FREITAS et al., 2012).

Preventable and non-preventable infant deaths are sentinel events and are linked to the fact that they could have been prevented by adequate health care. Preventable causes that can be reduced by adequate care for women during pregnancy and childbirth account for 46.6 per cent of neonatal deaths. This suggests the existence of problems in relation to maternal and child care, and indicates the need for greater investment to prevent and reduce neonatal deaths as a result of inadequate healthcare provision during pregnancy and after birth (ROCHA et al., 2011; FERNANDES et al., 2013).

Knowledge of the determinants of IM is an important tool for analysing the health situation of a region and can help evaluate programmes in the epidemiological surveillance of health problems, as well as guiding the identification of population groups most at risk of falling ill (FRIAS et al., 2010).

In Ceará, there is still a lot to be done in terms of infrastructure and actions directly aimed at pregnancy, childbirth and puerperium care, in order to improve mortality indicators at this stage of life (BEZERRA-FILHO et al., 2007).

Considering the magnitude of the occurrence of a child death for the family and society, and that most of these deaths could have been preventable, it is necessary to study the epidemiological profile of this type of mortality in order to know the main factors that influence the occurrence of death. Thus, this study is an extract from the Dissertation of
Sanders (2013) aimed to analyse the epidemiological profile of infant mortality in the municipality of Fortaleza - CE, between 2005 and 2010.

METHODS

This is a cross-sectional, quantitative and descriptive study carried out in Fortaleza - CE, between 2005 and 2010. It was carried out using secondary data from the Live Birth Certificates (DNV) and Death Certificates (DO) that feed the Live Birth Information System (SINASC) and the Mortality Information System (SIM).

The study population consisted of all deaths in children under one year old

(3,694) recorded in the DCs, made available by the Epidemiological Surveillance Cell (CEVEP) of the Fortaleza Municipal Health Department.

The study sample was selected by convenience on a non-probabilistic basis and consisted of 147 deaths. The aim was to select DCs with as much information as possible for the sample, and to select the deaths within the study period in an equitable manner. This justifies not analysing the entire population due to the lack of information in most of the fields (variables) of SINASC and SIM.

Data was collected at the CEVEP of the Municipal Health Department of Fortaleza, using a structured form with information on specific variables related to the characteristics of children under one year of age who died, as well as the characteristics of the mother, pregnancy and labour.

In order to identify deaths in children under one year old, the linkage technique was used to cross-reference the SINASC and SIM databases, using the Reclink software, with the following variables: number of DNVs, child's date of birth, birth weight, mother's home address and mother's name to identify the perfect match (DUPONT; PLUMMER, 2009).

The Statistical Package for the Social Sciences (SPSS) programme, version 18.0, was used to process the data. The general data was analysed descriptively using frequencies (simple and percentage) for the qualitative variables and parametric measures (mean and standard deviation) for the quantitative variables. The results were presented in tabular form and discussed in accordance with the relevant literature.

This study complied with the recommendations of Resolution 466/2012, **which regulates "research involving human beings" of the** National Health **Council** (BRASIL, 2012). It was submitted to and approved by the Research Ethics Committee of the State University of Ceará (UECE), under opinion No. 12446.

RESULTS

In Fortaleza, from 2005 to 2010, 230,080 live births were registered on the SINASC and 3,694 deaths in children under one year old were registered on the SIM. Of this total, 802 deaths occurred in 2005, 701 in 2006, 590 in 2007, 574 in

2008, 589 in 2009 and 438 in 2010.

Table 1 shows the distribution of infant mortality rates (IMR) and their components: neonatal mortality rate (NMR) and post-neonatal mortality rate (PNMR), from 2005 to 2010. All mortality rates fell over the years, except for 2009, which showed a slight increase on the previous year.

Table 1: Distribution of IMR, NMR and MMR per 1,000 live births in Fortaleza-CE between 2005 and 2010.

Year	TMI (%)	TMN (%)	TMPN (%)
2005	20,6	13,5	7,1
2006	17,3	11,3	6,0
2007	15,6	10,6	5,0
2008	14,8	9,9	4,9
2009	15,6	11,0	4,6
2010	11,9	8,1	3,8

Source: SMS/CEVEP/SIM/SINASC

As can be seen in Table 2, of the 147 deaths in the sample studied, the majority, 88 (59.9%), occurred in the early neonatal period (0 to 6 days), i.e. in the first week of life, with the main cause of death being preventable deaths, with 120 (81.7%) cases.

Table 2: Total deaths in children under one year old and their classification according to the Brazilian List of Avoidable Deaths, Fortaleza-CE, 2005 to 2010.

	N	%
Death		
Early neonatal	88	59,9
Late neonatal	31	21,1
Post-neonatal	28	19,0
TOTAL	147	100,0
Causes of death		
Avoidable causes	120	81,7
Ill-defined causes	04	2,7
Non-preventable causes (other causes of death)	23	15,6
TOTAL	147	100,0

According to table 3, of the preventable causes, the most prevalent were: infections specific to the neonatal period (25.0%), newborn respiratory distress syndrome (17.5%), prematurity and low birth weight (12.5). The majority of deaths were related to adequate care for women during pregnancy, with a total of 55 (45.8%) of the causes of death, followed by adequate care for the newborn, with 37 (30.8%) deaths.

Table 3: Classification of avoidable causes of death, according to the Brazilian List of

Avoidable Deaths, Fortaleza-CE, 2005 to 2010.

Classification of preventable causes	N	%
Immunisation actions	01	0,8
Adequate care for women during pregnancy		
Prematurity and low birth weight	15	12,5
Respiratory distress syndrome in newborns	21	17,5
Maternal conditions affecting the foetus or NB	07	5,8
Maternal pregnancy complications that affect the foetus or RN	12	10,0
Adequate care for women in labour		
Intrauterine hypoxia	02	1,8
Neonatal asphyxia	07	5,8
Neonatal aspiration	01	0,8
Complications of labour and childbirth	04	3,4
Adequate care for NBs		
Respiratory and cardiovascular disorders specific to the neonatal period	07	5,8
Infections specific to the neonatal period	30	25,0
Diagnosis and treatment actions	12	10,0
Health promotion actions	01	0,8
TOTAL	120	100,0

The average age of the mothers was 25.9 ± 6.5 years, with the minimum and maximum values being 14 and 42 years, respectively. The majority, 102 (69.4%) of the mothers, were aged between 20 and 34; 99 (67.3%) lived without a partner; 131 (89.1%) had less than 4 years of schooling; 131 (89.1%) had twin pregnancies; almost half, 74 (50.3%) had between 4 and 6 antenatal appointments; the vast majority, 138 (93.9%) had pregnancies of less than 37 weeks, i.e. the babies were born prematurely. The average birth weight was 2038.08 ± 350.09g, with a minimum of 370g and a maximum of 3850g, the vast majority of which were 140 (95.3%) weighing less than 2500g. As for gender, there was a higher prevalence of 81 (55.4%) males.

Table 4: Epidemiological profile of Óbidos according to the variables studied. Fortaleza-CE, 2005 to 2010.

Epidemiological variables	N*	%
Socio-demographic and socio-economic variables		
Age (years)		
< 20	27	18,4
20 a 34	102	69,4
>35	18	12,2
Marital status		
No mate	99	67,3
With a mate	48	32,7
Schooling (years of study)		
< 4	131	89,1

4 a 7	5	3,4
>8	7	4,8
Pregnancy and childbirth variables		
Type of pregnancy		
Unique	15	10,2
Twin	131	89,1
No. of consultations		
<3	26	17,7
4 a 6	74	50,3
>7	47	32,0
Weeks of pregnancy		
< 36 weeks	138	93,9
37 to 41 weeks	6	4,1
Type of labour		
Vaginal	141	95,9
Caesarean section	5	3,4
Sex of the child		
Male	81	55,4
Female	66	44,6
Birth weight		
<1500g	6	4,1
1500 to 2499g	134	91,2
> 2500g	6	4,1

* Values lower than the total sample due to missing answers on the DNV and DO.

DISCUSSION

Various studies have shown that improvements in the population's living conditions have led to reductions in infant mortality rates (IMR) in Brazil and around the world, especially in the post-neonatal component. In our study, in only one year, 2009, was there a slight increase in IMR, represented by the early neonatal component, while the others remained in decline as shown in various studies (HERNANDEZ et al., 2011; ALKEMA et al., 2014; PIZZO et al., 2014; BATISTA and CRUZ, 2015). Another study found similar data regarding avoidability, with 71.6% of deaths in the 2000/2001 cohort and 65.5% of deaths in the 2007/2008 cohort considered avoidable by SUS interventions. In the two biennia studied, infant mortality was concentrated in the early neonatal period and the majority of deaths were considered avoidable, especially due to adequate care for women during pregnancy (SANTOS et al., 2014).

A study on neonatal mortality found that the possible predictors of neonatal death are: Apgar score less than 7 at the 5th minute of **life, gestational age (< 32, 33-36 and > 37 weeks, low birth weight,** multiple births, use of mechanical ventilation at any time after birth, use of supplementary oxygen after birth, admission to a neonatal intensive care unit, use of continuous positive airway pressure, intubation in the delivery room, cardiac massage, drugs for resuscitation, phototherapy in the first 72 hours of life, use of surfactant and administration of antibiotics in the first 48 hours of life, report of congenital malformation, convulsions, respiratory diseases of the newborn, hypoglycaemia or necrotising enterocolitis (SILVA et al., 2014).

In relation to hospital care, referrals with guaranteed assistance for high-risk births and the technological advances incorporated into the area of neonatal care, such as assisted breathing, the use of antenatal corticoids and surfactant, were other factors perceived as contributing to the reduction in infant mortality (BARBOSA and CUNHA, 2011; PIZZO et al., 2014). These measures are capable of further reducing neonatal mortality rates, especially since they were the ones that showed the smallest reductions in this study. These are therefore strategies and actions to be considered by managers and policies that seek to reduce IMR.

Studies show that the biggest challenge is still to reduce neonatal mortality, which accounts for the largest proportion of deaths in children under one year old and is the most significant component of infant mortality. This difficulty results from the complex relationship between the adverse conditions of the mother and the newborn, low social status and difficulty in accessing health care, all of which contribute to an increased risk of death. Unlike post-neonatal mortality, the reduction of which is often associated with better living conditions for the population (SILVA et al., 2014).

In several studies, maternal age and schooling are associated with infant mortality, and are particularly important because of their interrelationship with other factors associated with deaths under one year of age.

We found a high percentage of mothers aged between 20 and 34, a result that is consistent with other studies (MAIA et al., 2012; NASCIMENTO et al., 2012; NORONHA et al., 2012). It has been pointed out that the extremes of reproductive age form part of the largest set of factors associated with infant mortality, i.e. children of mothers under 20 and those over 35 are more likely to die as infants (LIMA, 2010; BRASIL, 2012; FRIAS and NAVARRO, 2013). However, despite the evidence, there is no consensus on the extent to which maternal age can explain adverse obstetric outcomes

(LIMA, 2010).

There was a higher percentage of infant deaths among children born to mothers with low levels of education, which is similar to the literature, since studies show a significant association between lower levels of education and death in children under one year old (MAIA et al., 2012; FRIAS and NAVARRO, 2013).

The occurrence of death was higher among women who reported not having a partner, which corroborates a national study that revealed a strong association of neonatal mortality in mothers with single marital status, living without a partner (OR:2.55; 95%CI: 1.81-3.58) (LANSKY et al., 2014). The participation of a partner enables a greater financial contribution, as well as emotional support for the mother and the newborn, reflecting greater security and support for the care of both (BRASIL, 2012).

Another variable that was found to have a higher proportion of deaths in the group studied was multiple pregnancies, which is in line with other studies (ZANINI et al., 2011; MAIA et al., 2012; LANSKY et al., 2014). This event is related to the fact that live births from twin pregnancies have a high incidence of prematurity and low birth weight, conditions associated with the risk of infant mortality (BRASIL, 2012).

This study found a higher number of deaths in children under one year of age among mothers with a low number of prenatal care visits. Attendance at prenatal consultations has been explained by some studies as an important cause related to pregnancy and childbirth care in reducing infant morbidity and mortality in Brazil (ZANINI et al., 2011; NASCIMENTO et al., 2012; NORONHA et al., 2012; LANSKY et al., 2014). A greater number of visits during prenatal care offers greater protection for the newborn, since more frequent monitoring of pregnant women leads to the detection and early intervention of risk situations (BRASIL, 2012).

There is a consensus in the literature that premature newborns are at greater risk of early neonatal mortality (ZANINI et al., 2011; NORONHA et al., 2012; FRIAS and NAVARRO, 2013; LANSKY et al., 2014), and this fact was in agreement with the present study, since a high rate of children born at less than 36 gestational weeks was demonstrated. In all regions of the country, prematurity followed by infections, congenital malformations and asphyxia/hypoxia have been the main determinants of neonatal deaths (FRIAS and NAVARRO, 2013).

The Nascer no Brasil survey, a national study, revealed a high neonatal mortality rate in newborns born to mothers with a gestational age below 37 weeks, indicating a rate of

19.5/1,000 live births in those with 33-36 weeks of gestation and 30.6/1,000 live births was the rate of parturients with equal to or less than 32 weeks of gestation (LANSKY et al., 2014).

Brazilian studies also associate higher infant mortality with caesarean section (ZANINI et al., 2011; FRIAS and NAVARRO, 2013). However, this study showed a higher frequency of vaginal deliveries in the deaths investigated, corroborating other studies (NORONHA et al., 2011; ZANINI et al., 2011; OLIVEIRA et al., 2013). The precise indication of caesarean section helps to reduce the number of deaths among newborns classified as being at risk (ZANINI et al., 2011). Other circumstances that may be related to this result are the poor quality of vaginal delivery care and distortions in the indication of the route of delivery, such as caesarean sections in low-risk pregnancies and normal deliveries in situations of high foetal risk (LOURENÇO et al., 2013).

The results of this study show that a higher proportion of the deaths investigated were among male children. Other studies have shown an increased risk for male newborns (ZANINI et al., 2011; CARNEIRO et al., 2012; NASCIMENTO et al., 2012; LANSKY et al., 2014). The explanation for the higher mortality in males may be associated with the fact that lung maturation occurs later in this sex, leading to a greater occurrence of respiratory problems for them (NASCIMENTO et al., 2012).

Low birth weight (less than 2,500g) in newborns is intrinsically associated with infant mortality (ZANINI et al., 2011; NASCIMENTO et al., 2012; NORONHA et al., 2012). With regard to birth weight, there was a greater predominance of low birth weight deaths, similar to the results of other authors (MAIA et al., 2012; OLIVEIRA et al., 2013; LANSKY et al., 2014). It should also be noted that when analysing the avoidability of infant death, birth weight should be taken into account, since it is the single most important factor for infant survival (JACINTO et al., 2013).

CONCLUSION

It was concluded that the epidemiological profile of the deaths was characterised by young mothers, living without a partner, low levels of education, twin pregnancies, gestational age of less than 36 weeks, vaginal delivery and low birth weight of the newborn.

The fact that only secondary data was used is considered a limiting factor in this study, as there was a lack of information on many variables, as well as duplicate records in the SIM and SINASC databases. However, this finding did not invalidate the final analysis and its results.

However, it is important to raise awareness among health professionals about the correctness and completeness of filling in live birth and death certificates, so that the information collected is reliable and reflects reality. This measure would increase the consistency and reproducibility of epidemiological surveys for planning health actions, thus contributing to a reduction in infant mortality.

REFERENCES

ALKEMA, L.; FENGQING, C.; DANZHEN, Y.; PEDERSEN, J.; SAWYER, C.C. National, regional, and global sex ratios of infant, child, and under-5 mortality and identification of countries with outlying ratios: a systematic assessment. **Lancet Global Health**, v.2, n.9, p.521-30, 2014.

BARBOSA, A.P.; CUNHA, A.J.L.A. Neonatal and paediatric intensive care in Rio de Janeiro State, Brazil: an analysis of bed distribution, 1997 and 2007. **Cadernos de Saúde Pública**, v.27, sl.2, p.S263-S271, 2011.

BATISTA FILHO, M.; CRUZ, R.S.B.L.C. Children's health in the world and in Brazil. **Revista Brasileira de Saúde Materno Infantil**, v.15, n.4, p.451-4, 2015.

BEZERRA-FILHO, J.G.; KERR-PONTES, L.R.F.S.; MINÁ, D.L.; BARRETO, M.L. Spatial distribution of infant mortality rate and main determinants in Ceará, Brazil, in the period 2000-2002. **Cadernos de Saúde Pública**, v.23, n.5, p.1173-1185, 2007.

BRAZIL. Ministry of Health (MS). Health Care Secretariat.
Department of Programmatic and Strategic Actions. Newborn health care: a guide for health professionals. Brasília: Ministry of Health (MS); 2011. Volume 1.

BRAZIL. Ministry of Health. Health Surveillance Secretariat.
Department of Health Situation Analysis. Health Brazil 2011: a

analysis of the health situation and surveillance of women's health. Brasília: Ministry of Health Publishing House, 2012.

BRAZIL. Resolution no. 466/12. On research involving human beings. Official Gazette of the Federative Republic of Brazil, Brasília, DF, 2012.

BRAZIL. Ministry of Health. Health Care Secretariat. Department of Strategic Programme Actions. High-risk pregnancy: technical manual. 5. ed. Brasília: Ministry of Health; 2012.

CARNEIRO, J.A.; VIEIRA, M.M.; REIS, T.C.; CALDEIRA, A.P. Risk factors for mortality of very low birth weight infants in the Neonatal Intensive Care Unit. **Revista Paulista de Pediatria**, v.30, n.3, p369- 376, 2012.

DUPONT, W.D.; PLUMMER, W.D. PS Power and sample size calculations. Version 3.0. [S. l.: s. n.], Jan. 2009.

FERNANDES, C.A.; VIEIRA, V.C.L.; SCOCHI, M.J. Infant mortality and avoidability classification: researching municipalities in the 15th health region of Paraná. **Revista Ciências Cuidado e Saúde**, v.12, n.4, p.752-759, 2013.

FREITAS, B.A.C.; GONÇALVES, M.R.; RIBEIRO, R.C.L. Infant mortality, according to avoidability criteria and components - Viçosa - MG, 19982010. **Pediatria Moderna**, v.48, n.6, p.237-45, 2012.

FRIAS, P.G.; PEREIRA, P.M.H.; ANDRADE, C.L.T.; LIRA, P.I.C.; SZWARCWALD, C.L. Evaluation of the adequacy of information on mortality and live births in the state of Pernambuco, Brazil. **Cadernos de Saúde Pública**, v.26, n.4, p.671-681, 2010.

FRIAS, P.G.; NAVARRO, L.M. Children: subjects of rights and their vulnerability. In: Bittencourt SDA, Dias MAB, Wakimoto MD (Orgs.). Maternal, infant and foetal death surveillance and work with mortality committees. Rio de Janeiro: EAD/Ensp, 2013. ch.3, p.91-133.

HERNANDEZ, A.R.; SILVA, C.H.; AGRANONIK, M.; QUADROS, F.M.; GOLDANI, M.Z. Trend analysis of infant mortality rates and their risk factors in the city of Porto Alegre, Rio Grande do Sul, Brazil, from 1996 to 2008. **Cadernos de Saúde Pública**, v.27, n.11, p.2188-96, 2011.

JACINTO, E.; AQUINO, E.M.L.; MOTA, E.L.A. Perinatal mortality in the municipality of Salvador, Bahia: evolution from 2000 to 2009. **Revista de Saúde Pública**, v.47, n.5, p.846-853, 2013.

LANSKY, S.; FRICHE, A.A.L.; SILVA, A.A.M.; CAMPOS, D.; BITTENCOURT, S.D.A.; CARVALHO, M.L.; et al. Birth in Brazil Survey: profile of neonatal mortality and evaluation of care for pregnant women and newborns. **Cadernos de Saúde Pública**, v.30, sl.1, p.S192-S207, 2014.

LIMA, L.C. Maternal age and infant mortality: null, biological or socioeconomic effects? Revista Brasileira de Estudos Populacionais, v.27, n.1, p.211-226, 2010.

LOURENÇO, E.C.; BRUNKEN, G.S.; LUPPI, C.G. Neonatal infant mortality: a study of preventable causes in Cuiabá, Mato Grosso, 2007. **Epidemiologia e Serviços de Saúde,** v.22, n.4, p.697-706, 2013.

MAIA, L.T.S.; SOUZA, W.V.; MENDES, A.C.G. Differentials in risk factors for infant mortality in five Brazilian cities: a case-control study based on SIM and SINASC. **Cadernos de Saúde Pública,** v.28, n.11, p.2163-2176, 2012.

NASCIMENTO, R.M.; LEITE, A.J.M.; ALMEIDA, N.M.G.S.; ALMEIDA, P.C.; SILVA, C.F. Determinants of neonatal mortality: a case-control study in Fortaleza, Ceará, Brazil. **Cadernos de Saúde Pública**, v.28, n.3, p.559-572, 2012.

NORONHA, G.A.; TORRES, T.G.; KALE, P.L. Analysis of infant survival according to maternal, pregnancy, labour and newborn characteristics in the 2005 birth cohort in the municipality of Rio de Janeiro-RJ, Brazil. **Epidemiologia e Serviços de Saúde**, v.21, n.3, p.419-430, 2012.

OLIVEIRA, A.R.R.; LERENA JUNIOR, J.C.; COSTA, M.F.S. Profile of newborn deaths in the delivery room of a maternity hospital in Rio de Janeiro, 2010-2012. **Epidemiologia e Serviços de Saúde**, v.22, n.3, p.501-8, 2013.

PIZZO, L.G.P.; ANDRADE, S.M.; SILVA, A.M.R.; MELCHIOR, R.; GONZÁLEZ, A.D. Infant mortality in the perception of health managers and professionals: determinants of its decline and current challenges in a municipality in southern Brazil. **Saúde e Sociedade**, v.23, n.3, p.908-18, 2014.

ROCHA, R.; OLIVEIRA, C.; SILVA, D.K.F.; BONFIM C. Mortality and Avoidability: An Analysis of the Epidemiological Profile. **Revista de Enfermagem** UERJ, Rio de Janeiro, v.19, n.1, p.114-20, 2011.

SANDERS, L.S.C. **Infant mortality: analysing risk factors in a capital city in the Brazilian Northeast.** Fortaleza, 2013. 101f. Dissertation (Master's in Collective Health) - Health Sciences Centre, State University of Ceará, 2013.

SANTOS, H.G.; ANDRADE, S.M.; SILVA, A.M.R.; MATHIAS, T.A.F.; FERRARI, L.L.; MESAS, A.E. Preventable infant deaths by interventions of the Unified Health System: comparison of two birth cohorts. **Ciências e Saúde Coletiva,** v.19, n.3, p907-16, 2014.

SILVA, A.A.M.; LEITE, A.J.M.; LAMY, Z.C.; MOREIRA, M.E.L.M.; GURGEL, R.Q.; CUNHA, A.J.L.A, et al. Neonatal near miss morbidity in the Nascer no Brasil survey. **Cadernos de Saúde Pública**, v.30, sl.1, p.S182-S191, 2014.

ZANINI, R.R.; MORAES, A.B.; GIUGLIANI, E.R.J.; RIBOLDI, J. Contextual determinants of neonatal mortality in Rio Grande do Sul using two analysis models. **Revista de Saúde Pública,** v.45, n.1, p.79-89, 2011.

CHAPTER 7

PROFILE OF OPIOID USE IN A NEONATAL INTENSIVE CARE UNIT

Regina de Carvalho Kinjo
Rôsicler Pereira de Gois
Francisco José Maia Pinto
Thamyres Fortaleza Monteiro
Rafaella Maria Monteiro Sampaio

INTRODUCTION

Pain relief and patient comfort are primary medical missions, involving ethical and humanitarian issues in the practice of medicine, and so the pain of the newborn must also be recognised and treated (GUINSBURG, 1999).

The development of neonatal intensive care units has led to a reduction in the mortality of critically ill newborns, whether premature or not. At the same time as the sophistication of therapeutic resources, a greater number of tests and invasive procedures are necessary to guarantee the survival of these newborns. In other words, surviving the neonatal period comes at a cost to the patient, including pain (GUINSBURG, 1999).

Studies in the 1990s showed that a large number of health professionals know that newborn babies (NBs), even premature ones, are capable of feeling pain in a similar way, or even more intensely than adults, and that various procedures carried out in the Neonatal Intensive Care Unit (NICU) are painful, but even so, pain relief measures are not often employed (CASTRO et al., 2003; PRESTES et al., 2005).

Anand and Selanikio (1996), in an experimental study, confirmed the hypothesis that repeated exposure to pain in the neonatal period can cause permanent alterations or long-term changes, due to the development of plasticity in the immature brain, which can alter the pain system, associated with a decrease in the pain threshold during development; as well as greater vulnerability to stress and anxiety disorders as an adult.

Similar behavioural changes have been observed during infancy in newborns who have been exposed to prolonged periods of hospitalisation in Neonatal Intensive Care Units (NICUs) (AYMAR and COUTINHO, 2008). Despite this knowledge, almost 80 per cent of children admitted to NICUs are still under-treated. This may be related to a lack of knowledge of the anatomy and physiology of pain transmission, pain assessment scales, the pharmacokinetics and pharmacodynamics of analgesics, as well as insecurity in administering drugs to the neonatal population due to fear of adverse effects (KRAYCHETE et al., 2014).

As for pain therapy itself, non-pharmacological resources can be used, such as non-nutritive sucking of sugar water, as well as analgesics. The use of analgesics should be considered for all newborns with potentially painful diseases and/or undergoing invasive procedures, whether surgical or not (GUINSBURG, 1999). Among the group of non-opioid analgesics, only Paracetamol® is authorised for use in the neonatal period. However, in Brazil, there is no presentation for parenteral use, which limits its use in neonatal intensive care units. In addition, the onset of analgesic action is slow, around 1 hour, and it is not very effective in intense pain (GUINSBURG, 1999; AYMAR and COUTINHO, 2008).

Opioid analgesics are the most important weapon in the treatment of severe pain. They act through opioid receptors spread throughout the central nervous system, whose activation inhibits the transmission of the nocireceptive stimulus to the higher processing and association centres. Opioids inhibit pain afferents in the spinal cord and simultaneously activate descending cortical pain-inhibitory pathways, thus leading to analgesia. The interaction of these drugs with other types of opioid receptors triggers, in parallel to analgesia, respiratory depression, varying degrees of sedation, urinary retention, nausea, vomiting and physical dependence. The side effects that accompany opioid analgesia and sedation include respiratory depression, tolerance and physical dependence. Modern neonatal intensive care units have used opioids to relieve severe acute pain resulting from invasive procedures and surgeries (KRAYCHETE et al., 2014).

In Brazil, there is little research on the use of analgesia in neonatal intensive care units, as well as on medical education on the subject. In inpatient units, there is a gap in knowledge about how neonatal pain is perceived, the application of pain scales, non-drug analgesic procedures and low to high potency analgesic drugs that can be used for severe pain.

Thus, learning about pain and the therapeutic resources used to relieve it, especially analgesic drugs, contributes to the dissemination of knowledge that will only benefit critically ill neonates in neonatal units in the short and long term.

METHODS

An observational, cross-sectional and descriptive study carried out in a tertiary paediatric hospital (Hospital Infantil Albert Sabin/HIAS) from January to December 2014 (12 months) with all newborns admitted to the Neonatal Intensive Care Unit.

The information was taken from the unit's standardised indicator books, which monitor: number of patients admitted, length of hospital stay, main diagnosis, gender, gestational age, birth weight, age at admission, submission to mechanical ventilation, surgery, length of stay and outcome, as well as records of doses, adverse effects, use of the pain scale, drug weaning and application of risk scores.

The database was formatted in Epi-info 7.0, categorised according to the origin of the data. Univariate analyses were carried out using the SPSS statistical package. The research complied with the ethical aspects recommended by Resolution 466/12 of the National Health Council/Ministry of Health and was approved by the Research Ethics Committee of the Albert Sabin Children's Hospital.

RESULTS AND DISCUSSION

The sample comprised 100 newborns. There was an equivalence between the genders, with 50 per cent of the random sample being male and 50 per cent female; although the literature generally points to a greater susceptibility to illness among boys in various surveys (BORBA et al., 2014).

As can be seen in Table 1, 66 per cent of the neonates in the group were born at term, followed by 24 per cent who were moderately premature (between 32 and 36.6 weeks). The average gestational age was 36.6 weeks. As for birth weight, 55% of the patients weighed over 2500g, followed by 45% of low birth weight neonates. The average weight of the sample was 2570±147g. Of the 100 patients, 51 received a surgical diagnosis. Orotracheal intubation/mechanical ventilation was the most common painful procedure (91%).

Table 1: General characteristics of the 100 neonates using opioids in the neonatal ICU

Features	%
GESTATIONAL AGE	
25-31sem	10%
32-36sem	24%
37-42sem	66%
BIRTH WEIGHT	
1001-1500g	10%
1501-2499g	35%
2500-4500g	55%
DIAGNOSIS	
Clinical	49%
Surgical	51%
MECHANICAL VENTILATION	
Yes	91%
No	9%
TOTAL	**100%**

The SNAPPE II and NTISS neonatal severity scores were used to establish the clinical severity profile of these patients. The group's average score was 21 and 17 points respectively. In national neonatal ICUs, a SNAPPE II score higher than 24 is directly proportional to the number of early neonatal deaths (SILVEIRA et al., 2001; PROCIANOY and ZARDO, 2003). The most prevalent illnesses that led to hospitalisation were malformation (50), infection (16), heart disease (15) and asphyxia (10) (Graph 1).

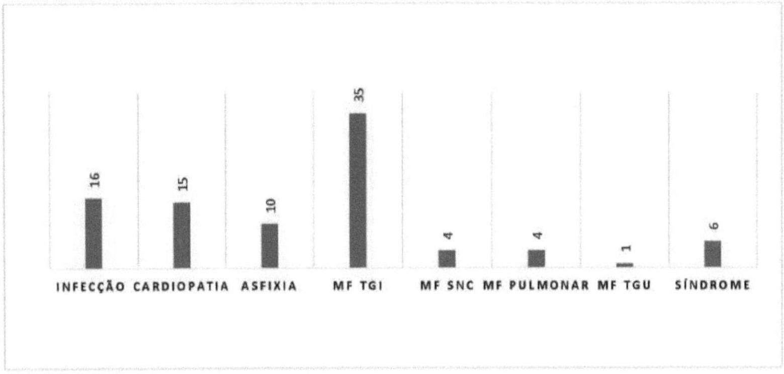

Graph 1: Most prevalent diagnoses.

All cases received opioid analgesia. A study led by Guinsburg et al. (2005) in university ICUs across the country showed that around 25% received some form of analgesia during hospitalisation. The main indications for powerful analgesia were: tracheal intubation, mechanical ventilation, agitation, post-surgery and pain (PROCIANOY and ZARDO, 2003). Simon et al. (2004) reported that among 1,375 patients admitted to the ICU up to 14 days old, only 15 to 32 per cent received some dose of analgesia. Anand and Selanikio (1996), when studying 109 ICUs in North America, reported an analgesia rate of 27 per cent in the first week of life for critically ill neonates (HARRISON et al., 2006; MAIA et al., 2011).

Among the clinical illnesses, complex heart disease and pulmonary hypertension under IMV received the most analgesia (23%). Necrotising enterocolitis led to analgesia in 5% of cases. Respiratory problems (air leak syndrome, respiratory distress syndrome and pulmonary hypertension) are the main indications for sedoanalgesia in ICUs (CASTRO et al., 2003; GUINSBURG et al., 2005).

In the current study, the routine application of the standardised Pain Scale (CRIES and NFCS) was offered to 62% of the cases. The scales were applied in all post-operative periods at intervals of 2/2 hours on the 1st post-operative day and increasing the interval thereafter. Severe clinical illnesses had their interval of assessment by the scales established at the doctor's discretion. Pain scales are still rarely used in ICUs, even in international services (HARRISON et al., 2006; CARBAJAL et al., 2008).

A literature review by Maia and Coutinho (2011) on recognising and dealing with pain in ICUs shows that health professionals are still predominantly concerned with: the lack of analgesic routine, unfamiliarity with pain scales and overestimating the subjective aspect of neonatal pain.

Mechanical ventilation is still the main indication for starting opioids in our country. Although 91% of the group underwent IMV, only 49% were intubated and given opioids. Among the patients intubated for IMV, around 28% continued with the prescribed analgesic drug. Data from the United Kingdom recorded that ICU professionals using analgesia before intubation grew from 37% in the mid-2000s to 71% today (SIMON et al., 2004).

In a study by Castro et al. (2003), 55% of NBs received analgesia after 24 hours of IMV, and agitation was the most common indication recorded in medical records. In agreement with other surveys, surgery or a painful procedure increased the indication for potent analgesia. Opioid analgesics were started after recovery from anaesthesia or an altered pain scale in all patients who underwent surgery (51%). In the general group, opioids were more commonly indicated after the 3rd day of hospitalisation (41%) for various reasons, especially the need for greater sedation. Analgesia for wound pain was recorded and medicated in 12% of patients. As in other studies, Fentanyl® was the most commonly used opioid (93%), followed by Tramadol®. There was a preference for the second drug when the patient was off IMV.

Fentanyl® is a potent, short-acting narcotic analgesic, 100 times more potent than morphine. It is indicated for induction of anaesthesia and treatment of severe pain. Depending on the dose given, analgesia lasts between 30 minutes and 6 hours. It can be administered intramuscularly or intravenously, intermittently or continuously (SILVA et al., 2007).

In newborns, it has a powerful analgesic effect at a dose of 2-5mcg/kg/h. It has fewer cardiovascular effects (bradycardia) than other analgesics, although it induces rapid tolerance. Doses higher than 3mcg/kg/min favour rib cage rigidity, hypotension and urinary retention. Its most feared side effect is respiratory depression.

For this group, opioids were initially prescribed at a dose of 1mcg/kg/min in continuous intravenous infusion for 56% of cases and then adjusted according to the pain scale. The average dose offered ranged from 1.4 - 2mcg/kg/min. Around 6% of patients exceeded the dose of 3.5mcg/kg/min. The average time opioid analgesics were given was 7.1 days (Table 2).

Table 2: Characteristics of opioid prescriptions in the neonatal ICU

Features	%
STARTING AGE	
0-1day	28%
2-3 days	28%
4-28days	41%
>28days	3%
INITIAL DOSE	
0.5 mcg/kg/h	4%
1 mcg/kg/h	56%
2 mcg/kg/h	37%
3 mcg/kg/h	3%
MAXIMUM DOSE	
0.5 mcg/kg/h	2%
1 mcg/kg/h	33%
2 mcg/kg/h	33%
3 mcg/kg/h	26%
4 mcg/kg/h	6%
TIME OF USE	
1 to 3 days	42%
4 to 7 days	31%
>8days	27%
TOTAL	**100%**

The study by Taddio (2002) identified signs of dependence after a cumulative dose of Fentanyl® of 1.6mg/kg to 2.5mg/kg or after 5-9 days of continuous infusion.

Tramadol ® is another narcotic analgesic of moderate potency (1/10 of morphine) that can be administered enterally, intramuscularly or intravenously. It has good analgesic power and a lower risk of respiratory depression than Fentanyl (SILVA et al., 2007). In this group, neonates with moderate pain, without serious metabolic alterations, difficult vascular access, side effects to Fentanyl and/or without invasive ventilatory support received intermittent analgesia with Tramadol. The dose was set at 1.5mg/kg/dose up to every 6 hours according to the pain scale. Only 4 patients were medicated in this way.

The administration of opioids was followed by monitoring of side effects. The most common side effects were bradycardia (36 per cent), tongue fasciculation (32 per cent) and urinary retention (11 per cent). No apnoea, paralytic ileus or rib cage rigidity were recorded. This can be explained by the careful management of the average doses offered, which rarely exceeded 3mcg/kg/hour. In the event of adverse reactions, the doses were reduced or the drug was replaced (Graph 2).

After 3 to 5 days of continuous opioid infusion, tolerance or withdrawal syndrome can occur. In neonates, the liposolubility of the drugs or the **low content of** a-1 acid glycoprotein (the protein to which the opioid normally binds) leaves a greater free fraction of opioid in the plasma. After taking the drug for more than three days, it should be gradually withdrawn in order to avoid withdrawal syndrome. 59% of patients were weaned off the drug, with a reduction of 0.5-1mcg/kg/hour every 12 or 24 hours.

In the sample evaluated, 5 per cent of NBs had withdrawal syndrome, defined by the clinical criteria of the Finnegan Scale. Among the most common symptoms are: tachycardia, agitation, sweating, nausea, vomiting, diarrhoea, sleep disorders and even rebound pain (FINNEGAN, 1986).

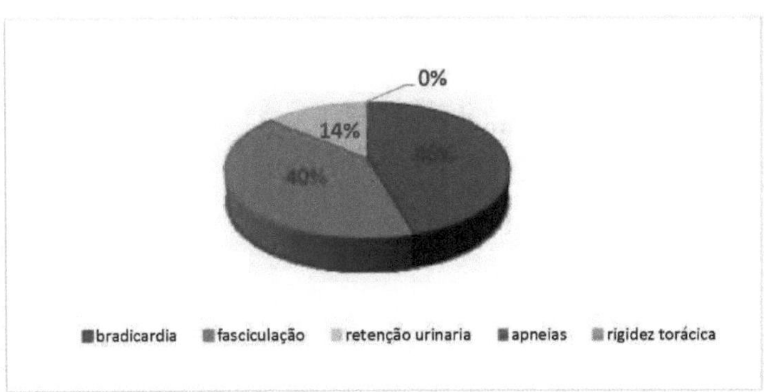

Graph 2: Adverse effects of opioids.

Avila-Alvarez et al. (2015) cited a 15.2% rate of withdrawal syndrome with the use of sedatives/analgesics in a European study. As no patient showed signs of withdrawal with the use of opioids for less than 3 days, the antagonist Naloxone® was not administered.

No patient was mediated with Morphine®. The service abandoned its use due to its slow onset of action, its low solubility, its delayed clearance in newborns, its hypotensive effect and bronchial reaction, its relationship with food intolerance and severe peri-intraventricular haemorrhage; as well as the risk of neuronal apoptosis and leukomalacia (SILVA et al., 2007; AVILA- ALVAREZA et al., 2015).

Following the unit's written routine, once the maximum dose of 3.5 to 4mcg/kg/hour had been reached and the necessary sedation was not achieved, another drug should be added. The benzodiazepine Midazolam® was the main choice in 13% of cases, especially in patients with severe pulmonary hypertension and post-operative correction of oesophageal atresia with fistula. The dose of Midazolam® ranged from 0.01 to 0.05mcg/kg/h. No premature babies received Midazolam®.

Around 71 were discharged from hospital. The average length of stay was 19.2 days, and 57 per cent were discharged before 15 days of life. The pain-mortality relationship has already been studied by several researchers who link the release of catecholamines and cortisol to severe suffering. Hyperglycaemia and lactic acidosis are strong markers of painful stress. Neonates with severe illnesses, without analgesia or with sub-therapeutic doses are more likely to suffer from bleeding, higher oxygenation rates on IMV, infections, neurological disabilities and death (EVANS et al., 2000; ARANDA et al., 2005).

CONCLUSION

The use of opioid analgesics in Neonatal Intensive Care Units requires knowledge of the peculiarities of neonatal pain, its objective measurement using standardised scales, the choice of safe drugs and the monitoring of adverse effects.

In a population of critically ill neonates, analgesia is still indicated before tracheal intubation and mechanical ventilation, although progress has been made in relieving pain and the complications of other serious and painful illnesses. Fentanyl proved to be a safe drug when used under 3mcg/kg/hour continuously and for less than 3 days. However, monitoring for signs of withdrawal needs to be improved.

REFERENCES

ANAND KJS, SELANIKIO JD, SOPAIN study group. Routine analgesic practice in 109 neonatal intensive care units. **Paediatr Res**, v.39, p.192A, 1996.

ARANDA JV, et al. Analgesia and sedation during mechanical-ventilation in neonates. **Clinical Therapeutics,** v.27, p.877-99, 2005.

AVILA-ALVAREZA A, CARBAJALB R, COURTOISB E, PERTEGA-DIAZC S, MUNIZ-GARCIAD J, ANANDE KJS. Spanish Group of the Europain Project. Sedation and analgesia practices among Spanish neonatal intensive care units. **An Pediatr (Barc)**, v.83, n.2, p.75-84, 2015.

AYMAR CLG, COUTINHO SB. Factors related to the use of systemic analgesia in neonatology - review article. **Revista Brasileira de Terapia Intensiva**, v.20, n.4, p.405-410, 2008.

BORBA, GG, NEVES ET, ARRUÉ AM, SILVEIRA A, ZAMBERLAN KC. Factors associated with neonatal morbidity and mortality: a review study. **Saúde**, Santa Maria, v.40, n.1, p.09-14, 2014

CARBAJAL R, ROUSSET A, DANAN C, et al. Epidemiology and treatment of panful procedures in neonates in intensive care units. **JAMA**, v.300, p.60-70, 2008.

CASTRO MC, GUINSBURG R, ALMEIDA MF, PERES CA, YANAGUIBASHI G, KOPELMAN BI. Profile of the indication for opioid analgesics in newborns on mechanical lung ventilation. **Jornal de Pediatria**, v.79, p.41-8, 2003.

EVANS DJ, et al. Neonatal catecholamine levels and neurodevelopmental outcome: a cohort study. **Arch Dis Child Fetal Neonatal**, v.84, p.F49-F52, 2000.

FINNEGAN LP. Neonatal abstinence syndrome: assessment and pharmacotherapy, in: Neonatal Therapy: an update. Excerpta Medica, 1986;122-146.

GUINSBURG, R. Evaluation and treatment of pain in the newborn. **Journal of Paediatrics**, v.75, n.3, p.149-60, 1999.

GUINSBURG R, PRESTES AC, BALDA RC, MARBA ST. Frequency of analgesic use in university neonatal intensive care units. **Jornal de Pediatria,** v.81, n.5, p.450-10, 2005.

HARRISON D, LOUGHNAN P, JOHNSTON L. Pain assessment and procedural pain management practises in neonatal units in Australia. **Journal of Paediatrics and Child Health,** v.42, p.6-9, 2006.

KRAYCHETE DC , SIQUEIRA JTT, GARCIA JBS. Recommendations for opioid use in Brazil: Part II. Use in children and the elderly - Review article.
Revista Dor, v.15, n.1,2014.

MAIA AC, COUTINHO SB. Factors that influence the practice of health professionals in the management of newborn pain. **Revista Paulista de Pediatria**, v.29, n.2, p.270-6, 2011.

PRESTES AC, GUINSBURG R, BALDA RC, MARBA ST, RUGOLO LM, PACHI PR, et al. Frequency of analgesic use in university neonatal intensive care units. **Jornal de Pediatria**, v.81, p.405-10, 2005.

PROCIANOY RS, ZARDO MS. Mortality risk scores in neonatal ICUs. **Revista de Saúde Pública**, v.37, n.5, p.591-6, 2003.

SILVA YP, GOMEZ RS, MÁXIMO TA, SILVA ACS. Sedation and analgesia in Neonatology. **Revista Brasileira de Anestesiologia**, v.57, n.5, p.575-587, 2007.

SILVEIRA RC, SCHLABENDORFF M, PROCIANOY RS. Predictive value of SNAP and SNAP-PE scores in neonatal mortality. **Jornal de Pediatria,** v.77, p.4455-60, 2001.

SIMON L, et al. Premedication for tracheal intubation: a prospective survey in 75 neonatal and paediatric intensive care units**. Critical Care Medicine**, v.32, p.565-568, 2004.

SIMONS SHP, DIJK MV, LINGEN RAV, ROOFTHOOFT D, et al. Routine morphine infusin in preterm newborns who received ventilatory support: a randomised controlled trial. **JAMA**, v.290, p.2419-27, 2003.

TADDIO A. Opioid analgesia for infants in the neonatal intensive care unit. **Clin Perinatol**, v.29, p.493-509, 2002.

CHAPTER 8

CRITERIA FOR THE INDICATION OF PACKED RED BLOOD CELLS IN A NEONATAL INTENSIVE CARE UNIT

Vinícius Ramalho Dantas Araújo

Rôsicler Pereira de Gois

Francisco José Maia Pinto Mara Iza

Holanda de Almeida Rafaella Maria

Monteiro Sampaio

INTRODUCTION

The transfusion of blood components and blood derivatives is part of the therapeutic arsenal that provides advanced support for babies at risk in neonatal intensive care units. Newborn babies (NB) are the group of patients who consume the most blood and blood components in paediatric hospitals. The lower their weight and gestational age, the greater the need for transfusion (DINIZ et al., 2001).

As more and more immature newborns are surviving, the issue of anaemia, the repercussions of transfusion treatment and, in particular, the adoption of a policy to reduce blood transfusions have become huge challenges. Preterm infants with gestational ages <30 weeks, birth weights <1,000 g and those with severe infectious diseases are the main candidates for blood transfusions (ZUPPA et al., 1995).

There are many reasons why anaemia occurs in neonates. In the delivery room, early cord ligation and perinatal placental losses reduce haematological indices. However, the main reason for the high frequency of anaemia among newborns is iatrogenic: the excessive collection of samples required for laboratory tests (ALBIERO et al., 1998). Other causes in the neonatal period are late premature anaemia, occult bleeding, insufficient red cell production, surgical losses and haemolysis (GUEDES et al., 2004).

NB with respiratory failure, on oxygen therapy or mechanical ventilation, with bronchopulmonary dysplasia, apnoea or irregular respiratory rhythm, have higher oxygen demands and may benefit from the transfusion of small volumes of packed red blood cells (PRBC) (ALBIERO et al., 1998).

Defining normal haematometric indices in the neonatal period is particularly difficult. The variation in these values, which are considered normal in the full-term newborn, generally does not apply to the premature newborn, and can be different in the low birth weight and extreme low birth weight newborns. The haematocrit (Ht) values, haemoglobin (Hb) concentration and number of erythrocytes obtained in the newborn vary according to the nature of the vascular source, being 5 to 25 % higher in capillary blood (GUEDES et al., 2004). In addition, the association between necrotising enterocolitis and retinopathy of prematurity generated by transfusions of packed red blood cells (PRBCs) has been reported in the literature (BENNETT-GUERRERO et al., 2007; REYNOLDS et al., 2007).

Several strategies have been proposed to reduce the number of blood component transfusions in neonatology: avoiding prematurity, scheduling cord clamping within 2 minutes of birth, limiting blood collections, opting for micro-collections, reinforcing non-invasive monitoring, using restrictive transfusion criteria and rationalising the indications for human erythropoietin. International criteria for indicating haemotransfusion provide guidance on volume and underlying clinical conditions (OHLS, 2000) (Chart 1).

Table 1: Criteria for the indication of packed red blood cells

Hb (g/dl) / Ht (%)	**Mechanical Ventilation / Symptomatology**	**Red blood cell concentrate**
Hb< 13 / Ht< 40	In the first 24 hours of life (anaemia due to acute / subacute loss)	15ml/kg (2-4 hours)
Hb<11 / Ht<35	Moderate or significant MV (MAP > 8cm H2O and FiO2 > 0.4)	15 ml/kg (2-4 hours)
Hb<10 / Ht<30	Minimum MV (any MV or CPAP > 6cm H2O and FiO2 < 0.4)	15 ml/kg (2-4 hours)
Hb<8 / Ht<25	Absence of MV but one or more of the following criteria: *Tachycardia (>180/min) or tachypnoea (>80/min) >24h *FiO2 > 4x the FiO2 of the previous 48h by nasal cannula or CPAP >21% that of the previous 48h *Weight gain <10g/kg/day in the previous 4 days, receiving >100kcal/kg/day *Increased episodes of apnoea and bradycardia, despite therapeutic doses of methylxanthines (> 10/24h or > 2 episodes/24h requiring ambu) *Submitted to Surgery	20 ml/kg (2-4 hours) Divide into 2 of 10ml/Kg)
Hb£7 / Ht<20	Asymptomatic and absolute **reticulocyte** count **<100,000cel/pl**	20 ml/kg (2-4 hours) Divide into 2 of

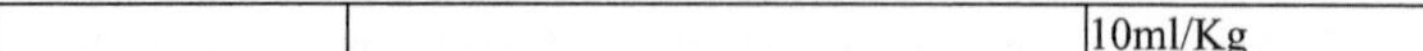

		10ml/Kg

Platelet concentrate is the second most requested type of blood component in neonatology. This blood component is used to treat haemorrhages caused by or accompanied by a reduction in the number and/or function of platelets. Thrombocytopenia in the neonatal period can affect 25 to 40 per cent of neonates admitted to neonatal intensive care units and 0.2 per cent of presumably normal neonates in the nursery. The criteria for platelet infusion are already well defined in clinical practice (STRAUSS, 2000).

Transfusion of fresh frozen plasma (FFP) is infrequent in the neonatal age group. FFP is indicated above all for the replacement of vitamin K-dependent factors (II, VII, IX, X, protein C and protein S), in NB with prolonged prothrombin time and active bleeding, in those requiring emergency surgery and in disseminated intravascular coagulation (DIC) (HILLYER; BERKMAN, 1995).

Blood component transfusions can cause some immediate or delayed complications. A typical transfusion reaction involves fever, chills, tachydyspnoea, cyanosis, pruritus, erythema, hyper- or hypotension, pain, among other signs. Although the appearance of immediate post-transfusion reactions such as non-hemolytic febrile and urticarial reactions is not common in NB, these patients can present the phenomenon of reactional hyperinsulinemia and hypoglycaemia. NBs are also susceptible to post-transfusion syndrome, especially when polytransfused, but this is a benign syndrome characterised by transient maculopapular erythema, eosinophilia and thrombocytopenia (KABRA, 2003).

While controversy persists in neonatology over the restrictive or permitted transfusion of red blood cells, each service uses different routines and finds different clinical results, especially in terms of morbidity and mortality. It is essential to be familiar with the latest medical positions on the subject and compare them with the results and practices of each service in order to offer quality medicine to the critically ill newborn being treated in neonatal ICUs.

METHODS

This was an observational, cross-sectional and descriptive study carried out in a tertiary paediatric hospital (Hospital Infantil Albert Sabin/HIAS) between January and

December 2014 (12 months).

All newborns admitted to the Neonatal Intensive Care Unit of the Albert Sabin Children's Hospital (CETINE) who had received a blood transfusion took part in the study. The inclusion criterion was the prescription of packed red blood cells. Patients who received other blood components and not packed red blood cells were excluded.

The information was taken from the unit's standardised indicator books, which monitor: number of patients admitted, length of hospital stay, main diagnosis, gender, gestational age, birth weight, age at admission, submission to mechanical ventilation, surgery, length of hospital stay and outcome, as well as records of the number and type of blood components administered.

The database was formatted in Epi-info 6.04 and categorised according to the origin of the data (DNV/DO and hospital records).

Univariate analyses were carried out using the SPSS statistical package. The research complied with the ethical aspects set out in Resolution 466/12 of the National Health Council/Ministry of Health and was approved by the Research Ethics Committee of the Albert Sabin Children's Hospital.

RESULTS AND DISCUSSION

During the one-year period, 54 patients were transfused in the Neonatal Intensive Care Unit (18% of patients). Data from national surveys estimate that more than 50% of neonates admitted to the ICU receive a transfusion during hospitalisation and the prevalence is higher in premature infants (up to 75%). Research by Beserra et al. (2014) showed that ICU patients always lead the way when it comes to transfusions, regardless of age group.

The sample showed a slight prevalence of males (51.9%), in agreement with the percentage and gender of other studies. The greater cardiorespiratory and immunological immaturity of males is already known in neonatology as an explanation for various morbidities that are more common in this sex (SEKINE et al., 2008; ROCCO et al., 2009).

With regard to gestational age, 60.4 per cent of those transfused were born at term. Although the average gestational age was lower (35.2 weeks). Among the premature babies, only 22.6 per cent were extremely premature. Data from the Brazilian Neonatal

Research Network indicate a greater risk of receiving a transfusion when the neonate weighs less than 1500g and has a conceptual age of less than 32 weeks. In Brazilian NICUs, the average number of red blood cell transfusions varied between 34 and 75%, with premature babies being the biggest recipients of blood (40 to 56%) (SANTOS and GUINSBURG, 2012).

Higher oxygen demands, respiratory diseases (respiratory distress syndrome and bronchodysplasia), persistence of foetal HB (very oxygen-hungry) up to 3 months, erythropoietin deficiency up to the 6th-8th week of life and early anaemia are pointed out as causes of the higher demand for red blood cells in this age group (NOMURA, 2006).

The average birth weight of the neonates in the sample was 2316 ± 762g. The smallest patient weighed 580g and the largest 4200g. Around 56% of the sample was classified as low birth weight.

A survey by Santos and Guinsburg (2012) found that 56% of those transfused in a neonatal ICU weighed less than 1500g and that the average number of transfusions could double as their weight dropped. Although there was no consensus on which haematocrit index required transfusion in very and extremely low birth weight neonates, those weighing less than 1000g or those with cyanotic heart disease were the most transfused in the first week of life. Normally, clinically stable NBs with a haematocrit greater than 30% and a haemoglobin greater than 10g/dl are not transfused. Those with lower haematocrit values but who are asymptomatic deserve individualised treatment, weighing up the risks and benefits (NOMURA, 2006).

The patients were admitted 40.4 per cent on the first day of life and 63.7 per cent cumulatively before 72 hours of life. When the Severity Scores were measured, the SNAPPE II and NTISS scored 26 and 18 points respectively in this group, a measure close to the general population of newborns admitted to the NICU in the period. In the group, 47 per cent registered more than 30 points on the SNAPP and 44 per cent more than 20 points on the NTISS.

Research by Silveira et al (2001) associated SNAP-PE scores greater than 24 points with a higher risk of complications and death before 7 days of life. Curan and Rosseto (2014) found an average NTISS of 14 points in the NICU and a score of 23 points linked to deaths. Several authors have long used prognostic scores to predict complications and early death among critically ill patients in neonatal ICUs

(RICHARDSON et al., 1998; DORLING et al., 2005) (Table 1).

The main illnesses that led to hospitalisation were: congenital malformations (38.9%), sepsis (27.8%), respiratory illnesses (18.5%), congenital heart disease (13%) and perinatal asphyxia (7.4%). These conditions are also the most common causes of neonatal hospitalisation according to data from DATASUS (BRASIL, 2016).

Data from national NICUs with 4899 transfused children showed that the main indications for red blood cell transfusion were anaemia (66%), bleeding (12%) and coagulation disorders (12%). A survey of NICUs in 8 Brazilian states shows that the diseases that most contribute to the risk of neonatal transfusion are: infection (OR 3.37), necrotising enterocolitis (OR 4.16) and pulmonary bleeding (OR 2.18). Apnoea of prematurity was ranked 4th among the indications (SANTOS and GUINSBURG, 2012).

Table 1: General characteristics of haemotransfused neonates in the neonatal ICU

Features	%
SEX	
Male	51,9%
Female	48,1%
GESTATIONAL AGE	
25-31sem	22,6%
32-36sem	17%
37-42sem	60,4%
BIRTH WEIGHT	
500-1000g	11,5%
1001-1500g	21,2%
1501-2499g	23,2%
2500-4500g	24,2%
DIAGNOSIS	
Clinical	63%
Surgical	37%
AGE OF ADMISSION	
0-1day	40,4%
2-3 days	23,1%
>3days	36,5%

Of the 54 neonates transfused with red blood cell concentrates (18.7% of those admitted to the ICU during the period), only 24 used the formal criteria standardised by the unit's routines. Mean airway pressure (MAP) above 8mmHg, multiple apnoeas and the need for a higher oxygen fraction (FiO2) led the indications. Several authors argue that a MAP of 6 to 8mmHg in a neonate under IMV and with FiO2 greater than 35% is indicative of increased tissue oxygen demand, even with a haematocrit close to 40-45%, since the predominance of foetal haemoglobin makes oxygenation difficult until around 3 months of life (CARCILLO and FIELDS, 2002). The rate of tissue oxygenation is difficult to measure before 12 weeks of age (VALETE and BARBOSA, 2008).

Respiratory failure and the need for mechanical ventilation was recorded in 70.4% of cases. Oxygen supply above 35% is an important criterion for guiding transfusions. In this group, 68.5 per cent had a high oxygen demand. The average FiO2 before transfusion was 53%. On the other hand, neonates under CPAP can tolerate a haematocrit of between 25-30% and haemoglobin of between 8 and 10g/dl, as long as the FIO2 is lower than 35-40%, there are no apneas or congenital heart disease (VALETE and BARBOSA, 2008). In this group, 8 patients under CPAP or halo were transfused due to apnoeas.

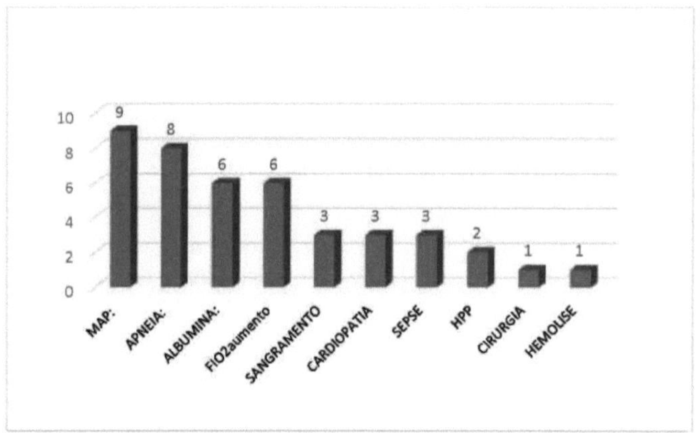

Graph 1: Criteria for red blood cell transfusion.

The association of anaemia with hypoalbuminaemia is quite common in severe, chronic or malnourished patients. Albumin is the most abundant protein in plasma (up to 60%) and plays an important role in transporting substances (e.g. bilirubin), maintaining oncotic pressure and tissue healing. Haemotransfusion prior to the supply of human albumin was justified by the known contraindication of infusing albumin in the presence of severe anaemia, which would represent a high risk of haemodynamic overload (CLOHERT et al., 2010).

In this sample, surgery was not an important cause for the indication of CH (1 indication), although 37% of the group had undergone surgery. Transfusions prior to surgical procedures are covered by various criteria (OHLS, 2000). Intra-operative transfusions, justified only in the event of significant blood loss (more than 20-25% of volemia) during the procedure, did not occur in this group; even given the NB's known low tolerance for acute blood loss (NOMURA, 2006).

The high metabolic demands of severe congenital heart disease are common reasons for indicating blood products, especially in cyanotic heart disease (high blood viscosity with low volume distribution) when a haematocrit above 40-45% is recommended. The justification is based on the fact that, physiologically, a haemoglobin concentration greater than 3g/dl is required to demonstrate clinical hypoxaemia/cyanosis (CLOHERT et al., 2010). In a group of 7 heart patients, only 3 of them received CH to maintain an adequate haematocrit. Furosemide was associated with CH in 53.7% of transfusions, which was justified by the risk of hypervolemia in a few cases.

Only one (1) patient received a red blood cell concentrate due to haemolysis. The indication was for persistent anaemia even after 2 blood transfusions due to Rh incompatibility and the risk of kernicterus. Haemolytic anaemia due to Rh or ABO incompatibility or G6PD deficiency was the leading indication for blood products in times before high-resolution phototherapy. Today it is restricted to a few cases that persist with positive direct Coombs and anaemia with symptoms. A red blood cell concentrate can be recommended even before exsanguineotransfusion if there is haemodynamic decompensation. It should be remembered that haemolysis due to irregular antibodies is rare even in polytransfused infants, a fact related to the relative incompetence of the NB's cellular immunity (DINIZ et al., 2001).

In 12 medical records, there was no explanation for the transfusion. These cases were classified as complying with liberal criteria for indicating CH, which place greater value on the clinical aspects of the patient and the experience of the professional following them. The combination of low haemoglobin with high oxygen demand or cardiac decompensation become common reasons for indicating haemotransfusion in these cases (CLOHERT et al., 2010).

Nopoulos et al. (2011) found a long-term reduction in white matter and subcortical nuclei in premature infants who received transfusions liberally. Whyte et al. (2009) found a score of less than 85 on the Bayley II neuropsychomotor development scale in children under 2 years of age who were given restricted transfusions in the neonatal period.

While adults are defined as maintaining haemoglobin greater than or equal to 10g/dl (to maintain saturation greater than 70% in the superior vena cava) in a situation of sepsis, there is no consensus in childhood. Paediatricians and neonatologists repeat this practice in order to maintain a good level of tissue oxygenation in the face of a severe systemic inflammatory reaction (RIVERS et al., 2001). In several studies, late-onset sepsis had the power to increase the indications for CH by almost 3 times; surpassing indications for coagulopathy, heart disease and surgery (FREITAS and FRANCESCHINI, 2012).

Transfusions were mostly indicated (73 per cent) before 15 days of life. Anaemia that starts before the second week of life is classified as early, while late anaemia occurs after the 6th-8th week. At the end of the 2nd or 3rd month of life, a haemoglobin level of 7-8g/dl is common and will soon be improved by the bone marrow's growing reaction to renal erythropoietin (VALETE and BARBOSA, 2008). The average age at transfusion was 12.2 days, despite the service's practice of scheduling the collection of tests.

Following the criteria cut-off points, 80.8% had a haematocrit of less than 30%. The average haematocrit before transfusions was 26.6%. FIO2 elevated beyond 35% was observed in 68.5%, with a mean supply of 53%. Clinical instability and uncontrolled sepsis contributed to indications for CH among patients with a haematocrit greater than 35%. The aliquot of 15ml/kg was preferred by intensivists in 48.1% of cases. The average volume prescribed was 16± 3ml/kg. A volume supply of 10ml/kg provides a yield of 3.g/dl of haemoglobin. To increase haemoglobin by 1g/dl, 3ml per kilo of red blood cell concentrate should be given in CPDA-1. Infusion of RBCs in a volume equal to or greater than 20 ml/kg can already generate volume overload. The volume to be given should be individualised (NOMURA, 2006).

Haemotransfusion was the only transfusion in 60.4% of patients and the average was 1.2 transfusions. The average number of transfusions in other NICUs varies between 1.6 and 5.9 transfusions per patient (SANTOS and GUINSBURG, 2012).

In Freitas and Franceschini's (2012) sample of premature babies, the median of 2 transfusions per patient applied to premature babies under 32 weeks with sepsis ($p=0.0001$).

In all infusions, the basic safety rules were followed: product at room temperature, infusion through exclusive access, compatible typing by cross-checking and infusion completed before 4 hours. Filtered and irradiated red blood cells were recommended for premature babies weighing less than 1200g (Table 2).

No cases of necrotising enterocolitis or retinopathy of prematurity appeared in this group after transfusion. However, some publications postulate the appearance of pro-inflammatory effects and the release of nitric oxide in the microcirculation (mesentery and retina) after haemotransfusion, which could increase the risk of enterocolitis and retinopathy. It is recommended to monitor enterocolitis in the first 48 hours after transfusion (MOHAMED and SHAH, 2012). No transfusion reactions were recorded during the period. In a study by Beserra et al. in another local tertiary hospital, 2.4% of reactions were recorded in the NICU, with fever being the most common sign and CH being the haemocomponent that generated the most reactions (BESERRA et al., 2014).

The practice of a single donor with immunocompatible blood extracted from a mother bag and fractionated into aliquots, although well practised in other units, was not common practice in this NICU. Unfortunately, the haematology service's routine of recommending that a new blood type be taken at every transfusion that was more than three days after the last sample must have contributed to the expulsion of neonates, despite the micro-collection. The practice of micro-collection associated with a single donor can reduce the number of transfusions in neonates by up to 50 per cent (BRASIL, 2010).

Table 2: Aspects of packed red blood cell transfusions in the neonatal ICU

Features	%
AGE AT TRANSFUSION	
<7days	36,5%
<14days	36,5%
<28days	19,2%
>29days	7,7%
TRANSFUSED VOLUME	
10ml/kg	15,4%
15ml/kg	48,1%
20ml/kg	36,5%
NUMBER OF TRANSFUSIONS	
1 transfusion	60,4%
2-3 transfusions	28,3%
>4transfusions	11,3%
HEMATOCRITE	
<20%	9,6%
<25%	21,2%
<30%	50%
<35%	19,2%

No cases of infection with cytomegalovirus, hepatitis B, hepatitis C or HTLV1 were recorded in this group. In Brazil, it is estimated that the risk of infection by these agents through a blood transfusion may be: 1% for cytomegalovirus, 1: 200mil for Hepatitis viruses and 1:3 million for HTL1 (ALLAIN et al., 2009). ANVISA recommends offering de-leucocytised products to polytransfused children to reduce the risk of infections by viral agents, especially cytomegalovirus and parvovirus (BRASIL, 2010).

The indication of recombinant human erythropetin (r-EPO) for the prevention of neonatal anaemia is not a consensus among neonatology services. When offered, r-EPO 250UI/kg subcutaneously or intravenously is given 3 times a week diluted in 5% human albumin and associated with Iron 4mg/kg orally or 1mg/kg parenterally. r-EPO has been shown to reduce the number of transfusions, but contributes to the generation of severe retinopathy (SANTOS and GUINSBURG, 2012). In this service, r-EPO is not routine. Among the sick neonates followed, 46.3% received an associated indication for other blood products, especially platelet concentrate.

When applying the X-test^2 with a 95% confidence interval, an association was found with a higher risk of CH transfusion for neonates weighing less than 1500g (p 0.0001), with a haematocrit of less than 25% (p 0.001) and undergoing surgery (p 0.0001). Length of hospitalisation over 23 days had an OR of 2.33.

The average length of hospitalisation for the group was 23 days. Around 52 per cent of neonates were hospitalised in the NICU for less than 15 days. In some studies, a hospital stay of more than 30-60 days can increase the risk of receiving a transfusion by up to 5 times (SANTOS and GUINSBURG, 2012). In this study, 55.6% of patients were discharged from hospital and 44.4% died.

CONCLUSION

The adoption of transfusion criteria helps to rationalise the number of transfusions in critically ill neonates and to respect their metabolic demands. The problem of early anaemia, accentuated by early ligation of the umbilical cord in the delivery room and excessive collection of tests, is still a serious problem that needs to be tackled. Premature and low birth weight neonates are still the biggest recipients of blood products.

REFERENCES

ALBIERO AL, DINIZ EMA, NOVARETTI MCZ, VAZ FAC, CHAMONE DAF. Transfusion of haemocomponents in term and premature NBs. **Revista da Associação Médica Brasileira**, v.44, p.201-9, 1998.

ALLAIN JP, STRAMER SL, CARNEIRO-PROIETTI AB, MARTINS ML, LOPES DA SILVA SN, RIBEIRO M, PROIETTI FA, REESINK HW. Transfusion-transmitted infectious diseases. **Biologicals**, v.37, p.71-7, 2009.

BENNETT-GUERRERO E, VELDMAN TH, DOCTOR A, TELEN MJ, ORTEL TL, REID TS, et al. Evolution of adverse changes in stored RBCs. **Proc Natl Acad Sci** USA, v.104, n.43, p.17063-8, 2007.

BESERRA MPP, PORTELA MP, MONTEIRO MP, et al. Transfusion reactions in an accredited hospital in Ceará: a haemovigilance approach. **Arq Med,** v.28, n.4, p.99-103, 2014.

BRAZIL. ANVISA. Resolution - RDC No. 57, of 16 December 2010.
Determines the Health Regulations for Services that develop activities related to the production cycle of human blood and components and transfusion procedures.
Available at:
http://bvsms.saude.gov.br/bvs/saudelegis/anvisa/2010/anexo/anexo_res0057_1 6_1 2_2010.pdf

BRAZIL. Ministry of Health. SUS Information Technology Department.
Health Indicators. Available at
http://www2.datasus.gov.br/DATASUS/index.php.

CARCILLO JA, FIELDS AI. Clinical practice parameters for haemodynamic support of paediatric and neonatal patients in septic shock. **Journal of Paediatrics**, v.78, n.6, 2002.

CLOHERT JP, EICHENWALD EC, STARK AR. Guidelines for common medications in the neonatal intensive care unit. In: Manual of Neonatology.
Editora Guanabara Koogan. 6th Ed. Rio de Janeiro. 2010, p544-54.

CURAN GRF, ROSSETO EG. Score system for neonatal therapeutic intervention: descriptive study. **Online Brazilian Journal of Nursing**, v.13, n.4, 2014.

DINIZ EMA, ALBIERO AL,CECCON MEJ, VAZ FAC. Use of blood, haemocomponents and haemoderivatives in the newborn. **Jornal de Pediatria,** v.77, sl.1, p.S104-14, 2001.

DORLING JS, et al. Neonatal disease severity scoring systems. **Arch Dis Chil Fetal Neonatal**, v.90, n.1, p.F11-6, 2005.

FREITAS BA, FRANCESCHINI SC. Factors associated with transfusion of packed red blood cells in premature infants in an intensive care unit.
Brazilian Journal of Intensive Care, v.24, n.3, p.224-9, 2012.

GUEDES MB, VASCONCELOS G, FRAGA G, PINTO R. Neonatal Anaemia - Transfusion Policy. Extract from

http://www.spp.pt/UserFiles/File/Consensos_Nacionais_Neonatologia_2004/ Neonatal_Anemia_Transfusion_Policy.pdf.

HILLYER CD, BERKMAN EM. Transfusion of plasma derivatives: fresh frozen plasma, cryoprecipitate, albumin and immunoglobulins. In: HOFFMAN R, BENZ EJ,

SHATTIL SJ, et al. Hematology - basic principles and practice. 2nd ed. New York: Churchill Livingstone; 1995. 2011-9.

KABRA NS. Blood transfusion in preterm neonates. **Arch Dis Fetal Neonatal Ed,** v.88, p.F38, 2003.

MOHAMED A, SHAH PS. Transfusion associated necrotising enterocolitis: a meta-analysis of observational data. **Paediatrics**, v.129, n.3, p.529-40, 2012.

NOMURA S. Blood transfusion in paediatrics: when and how much? In: LIMA CAVALCANTI I, DE FREITAS CANTINHO FA, ASSAD A, edl. Perioperative Medicine. Rio de Janeiro: SAERJ, 2006: 621-632.

NOPOULOS PC, CONRAD AL, BELL EF, STRAUSS RG, WIDNESS JA, MAGNOTTA VA, et al. Long-term outcome of brain structure in premature infants: effects of liberal vs restricted red blood cell transfusions. **Arch Pediatr Adolesc Med**, v.165, n.5, p.443-50, 2011.

OHLS RK. The use of erythropoietin in neonates. In: CHRISTENSEN RD. Neonatal haematology. **Clin Perinatol**, Philadelphia, WB Saunders Company, v.27, n.3, p.681-96, 2000.

REYNOLDS JD, AHEARN GS, ANGELO M, ZHANG J, COBB F, STAMLER JS. S-nitrosohemoglobin deficiency: a mechanism for loss of physiological activity in banked blood. **Proc Natl Acad Sci** USA, v.104, n.43, p.17058-62, 2007.

RICHARDSON DK, et al. Neonatal risk scoring systems. Can they predict mortality and morbidity? **Clin Perinatol**, v.25, n.3, p.591-611, 1998.

RIVERS E, NGUYEN B, HAVSTAD S, et al. Early goal-directed therapy in the treatment of severe sepsis and septic shock. **N Engl J Med**, v.346, p.1368-77, 2001.

ROCCO JR, SOARES M, ESPINOZA RA. Blood transfusion in intensive care: an observational epidemiological study. **Revista Brasileira de Terapia Intensiva**, v.18, n.3, p.242-50, 2006.

SANTOS AMN, GUINSBURG R. Why is it important to analyse factors associated with the indication of red blood cell transfusions in premature infants? **Revista Brasileira de Terapia Intensiva,** v.24, n.3, p.21-218, 2012.

SEKINE L, WIRTH LF, FAULHABER GAM, SELIGMAN BGS. Analysis of the profile of requests for blood component transfusions at the Hospital da Clínicas

in Porto Alegre in 2005. **Revista Brasileira de Hematologia e Hemoterapia**, v.30, n.3, p.208-12, 2008.

SILVEIRA RC, et al. Predictive value of SNAP and SNAP-PE scores in neonatal mortality. **Jornal de Pediatria**, v.77, p.4455-60, 2001.

STRAUSS RG. Blood banking and transfusion issues in perinatal medicine. In: CHRISTENSENS RD. Haematologic problems of the neonate. Philadelphia, WB

Saunders Company, 2000; 405-25.

VALETE CO, BARBOSA ADM. Blood transfusion for premature infants. **Pediatrics** (São Paulo), v.30, n.3, p.177-184, 2008.

VOLPATO SE, FERREIRA JS, FERREIRA VLPC, FERREIRA DC. Transfusion of packed red blood cells in the intensive care unit. **Revista Brasileira de Terapia Intensiva,** v.21, n.4, p.391, 2009.

WHYTE RK, KIRPALANI H, ASZTALOS EV, ANDERSEN C, BLAJCHMAN M, HEDDLE N, LACORTE M, ROBERTSON CM, CLARKE MC, VINCER MJ, DOYLE LW, ROBERTS RS. PINTOS Study Group. Neurodevelopmental outcome of extremely low birth weight infants randomly assigned to restrictive or liberal haemoglobin thresholds for blood transfusion. **Pediatrics**, v.123, n.1, p.207-13, 2009.

ZUPPA AA, MAZZOTTA M, MARAGLIANO G, GIRLANDO P, FLORIO MG, TORTOROLO G. Anaemia of prematurity: risk factors influencing red cell transfusions. **Minerva Pediatria**, v.47, n.1-2, p.13-8, 1995.

CHAPTER 9

ANALYSING CERVICAL CANCER SCREENING IN A HEALTH REGION

Elanny Cristina Pascôa Candeira

Katherine Jeronimo Lima

Fiama Kécia Silveira Teófilo

Radmila Alves Alencar Viana

Moacir Tavares Martins Filho

INTRODUCTION

Cervical cancer is an important health problem affecting the female population worldwide (WHO, 2014). In 2013, this disease ranked second among the most common types of cancer among women worldwide (WHO, 2013). Every year, around 266,000 women die from cervical cancer, with 87 per cent of these deaths occurring in low- and middle-income countries, and in developing countries this cancer is among the most frequent in the female population (WHO, 2014; INCA, 2015a).

In Brazil, cervical cancer is considered a priority in public health policies because of its high incidence, morbidity and mortality (THULER et al., 2012). According to estimates for 2016, the country will have 16,340 new cases, with an estimated risk of 15.85 cases per 100,000 women (INCA, 2015a).

For a decade (2003-2013), cervical cancer was among the three groups of cancers that most affected Brazilian women and even though there was a national screening programme, it was observed that the mortality rate from this disease did not fall (INCA, 2015b).

Mortality from cervical cancer is considered preventable, but at the same time, it has great potential for prevention and cure, due to its slow evolution through detectable and curable phases (DIAS et al., 2010; BRASIL, 2013a). In this case, if quality cytological screening is guaranteed, combined with appropriate treatment in the early stages of damage, it is possible to significantly reduce the incidence of cervical cancer, with a positive impact on morbidity and mortality rates (BRASIL, 2013; WHO, 2014; DERCHAIN et al., 2016).

Brazil's vast territory and the heterogeneous resources of local health services make it difficult to implement effective cervical cancer screening actions (KUSCHNIR, 2014). Furthermore, there is a correlation between incidence and mortality from cervical cancer in women with poorer living conditions, demonstrating a lack of social equity in access to cytopathological screening (BORGES et al., 2012; KUSCHNIR, 2014; DERCHAIN et al., 2016).

According to estimates for 2016, the state of Ceará has an incidence rate of 20.62 per 100,000 women for cervical cancer, which is high compared to the national rate of 15.85/100,000 and the average for the Northeast region of 19.49/100,000 for the same year (INCA, 2015a). It should also be noted that between 2006 and 2014, there was a 9.6 per cent increase in incidence estimates (INCA, 2014a). It is worth noting that it is the neoplasm with the highest incidence in the state after breast cancer.

The researcher's experience in the Public Health Residency allowed her to analyse the health situation in the state of Ceará. One of these was to assess the situation of cervical cancer in the state's health regions. Reflections emerged after verifying possible flaws in the monitoring and analysis of data from the Cervical Cancer Information System (SISCOLO) in the municipalities of the 16ª Health Region of Ceará. This led to the need for investigations into the situation of cervical cancer monitoring in the context of this Health Region.

Given the issues mentioned above, we recognise the importance of promoting studies that produce data and information on the situation of Cervical Cancer. In this way, they can draw up an epidemiological profile of the area studied and identify inequalities in screening coverage. Knowledge of these factors will help to plan more effective cervical cancer control strategies that are in line with the local needs of the female population. Given the issues mentioned above, we recognise the importance of promoting studies that produce data and information on the situation of cervical cancer follow-up.

The aim of this study is to analyse data from the Cervical Cancer Information System (SISCOLO) in the 16ª Health Region of Ceará - Camocim. It seeks to contribute to the implementation of planning actions and the definition of priorities aimed at tackling the disease in this region.

METHODS

This was a cross-sectional, descriptive study with a quantitative approach.

The setting for the research was the 16th Health Region of Ceará - Camocim, which is one of the 22 Health Regions that make up Ceará's healthcare model. The 16th Health Region is made up of the following municipalities: Barroquinha, Camocim, Chaval, Granja and Martinópole, according to the Regionalisation Master Plan - PDR/2014 (CEARÁ, 2014).

The region has a total population of 151,100 inhabitants, and the number of women of childbearing age (10 to 49 years) is 48,660 women. While the female population aged 25 to 64, the target audience for the cervical cancer prevention programme, is 81,061 women (BRASIL, 2010a).

For this study, the data analysed was primarily for women aged between 25 and 64, but a descriptive analysis was carried out on other age groups, such as those under 25 and over 64, living in the region studied and who were notified in the Cervical Cancer Information System (SISCOLO) database.

The information analysed corresponded to the years 2011 to 2014. The choice to start the period in 2011 comes from the fact that this is the year in which the age of women who undergo the Pap test was extended. Previously it was carried out on women aged between 25 and 59, but with the implementation of new national guidelines for cervical cancer screening, the age range was extended to 64 (INCA, 2011).

Secondary data was used from the databases of the Health Information System - Information System for the National Cervical Cancer Control Programme (SISCOLO) of DATASUS. Information was collected on cytopathological tests carried out in the SUS network between 01/01/2011 and 31/12/2014. The information was transferred to the TAB-WIM programme version 3.6b and then transferred to Excel 2013 where the spreadsheets for the databases were built.

This study analysed the following variables: the supply of the test, which was assessed using the indicator ratio of cytopathological tests to the target population; previous cytology time (how long ago, in years, the test was carried out); age group and type of alteration present in the test.

To analyse the alterations, the types of lesions were regrouped as described below:

- Atypia of Undetermined Significance of Cells (squamous atypia of undetermined significance, possibly non-neoplastic (ASC-US) + squamous atypia of undetermined significance when high-grade intraepithelial lesions cannot be ruled out (ASC-H) + atypia glandular cells (AGC);

- Low-grade intraepithelial lesion - LSIL;
- High-grade intraepithelial lesion - HSIL
- Invasive carcinoma;
- Adenocarcinomas (Adenocarcinoma ***in situ*** + Invasive adenocarcinoma).

After transferring the data obtained from the SISCOLO Information System to the TAB-WIM programme version 3.6b and Excel 2013, the data was analysed using descriptive statistics (proportions), using the TabWin programmes, version 3.6b. and Excel 2013.

Given that there was no direct contact with the women, since we used secondary data accessible from SISCOLO, available on the internet and therefore in the public domain, following Resolution 466/12, it was not necessary to pass the research through the Research Ethics Committee.

RESULTS AND DISCUSSION

According to information collected from SISCOLO, a total of 24,648 cytopathological tests were carried out between 2011 and 2014 in the 16ª Health Region of Ceará - Camocim.

The main and most widely used method for screening is the Pap test (cytopathological examination of the cervix), which carries out an initial classification between low-grade and high-grade lesions, defining the appropriate clinical approach (BRASIL, 2010b; INCA, 2011).

With regard to the ratio between cytopathological tests and the target population in the municipalities of the region, there has been an increase in the percentages over the years in the municipalities of the 16th Health Region of Ceará (Table 1).

This indicator refers to the ratio between the total number of tests carried out on women aged 25 to 64 and one third of the women in this age group living in the same place and period (INCA, 2014b). Although the municipalities have not yet reached the ideal parameter of 1 (one), according to the Ministry of Health's parameter, it can be seen that the figures presented showed significant variations during these four years, with an increase in the supply of preventive examinations.

Table 1: Ratio of cervical cytopathological tests in women aged 25 to 64 in the municipalities of the 16ª Health Region of Ceará- Camocim, 2011 to 2014.

Municipalities	2011	2012	2013	2014
Barroquinha	0,07	0,38	0.28	0,62
Camocim	0,09	0,61	0,82	0,91
Chaval	0,15	0,47	0,46	0,46
Farm	0,03	0,18	0,35	0,59
Martinopolis	0,13	0,55	0,72	0,92

Source: SISCOLO, 2015.

The results show an increase in the supply of the test in the period analysed, but this indicator has limitations, since it only assesses the supply of cytopathological tests according to the number of tests carried out and not the number of women examined, which does not show the real situation of coverage of the target population for screening. Another limitation of this indicator is the fact that it only reflects the population that undergoes cytopathological examinations in the SUS, and examinations carried out in supplementary healthcare are not counted, even though the total number of women in the ratio of examinations is calculated using these two groups of women.

Although this information reveals the capacity to offer the test, it needs to be analysed together with other variables such as previous cytology and the time of the previous cytology, in order to better verify the periodicity of the offer and the extent of the reach of the target population (DIAS et al., 2010).

Regarding the proportion of cytopathological tests according to age group, an average of 79% of tests were carried out on women aged 25 to 64, the target group for the cervical cancer prevention programme.

Table 2: Proportion of cervical cytopathological tests according to age group in the 16ª Health Region of Ceará-Camocim, 2011 to 2014.

	2011		2012		2013		2014	
Track Age	**N**	**%**	**N**	**%**	**N**	**%**	**N**	**%**
< 25 years	573	24,2	1.035	17,4	1.202	17,4	1.587	18,1
25-64 years	2.368	78,3	4.705	79,4	5.462	79,1	6.970	79,2
> 64 years	78	2,5	190	3,2	242	3,5	238	2,7
Total	3.019	100	5.930	100	6.906	100	8.795	100

Source: SISCOLO, 2015.

However, the results show that over 20.8 per cent of women underwent the test outside the age range recommended by the Ministry of Health in the period studied. This suggests the persistence of unnecessary diagnostic and therapeutic procedures. These results are similar to those of other studies (CARDOSO et al., 2014; SILVA et al., 2014).

Primary care has a fundamental role to play in getting to know its entire population, as well as identifying all women in the priority age group for cervical cancer prevention (BRASIL, 2013b). Stressing the importance of screening and health education actions to achieve wide coverage of cytopathological tests in the target population, enabling a significant reduction in incidence and mortality from cervical cancer (BRASIL, 2010b; SILVEIRA et al., 2015).

However, screening in Brazil is opportunistic, i.e. it is carried out when the woman seeks the health service (KUSCHNIR, 2014). In addition, primary care services do not have a population-based register of all the women in their area for screening, which prevents them from identifying women who need the test (BRASIL, 2013; KUSCHNIR, 2014; NAVARRO et al., 2015).

According to the data collected, with regard to the frequency of previous cytology, there was a prevalence of up to one year,

representing an average of 43.8% of the total carried out in the years evaluated. This was followed by the period of up to two years, with an average percentage of 26.3% (Table 3).

Table 3: Cytopathological examinations according to time of previous cytology in women aged 25 to 64 from the 16ª Health Region of Ceará-Camocim.

	2011		**2012**		**2013**		**2014**	
Period	**N**	**%**	**N**	**%**	**N**	**%**	**N**	**%**
Same year	113	4,6	202	4,3	207	4	313	4,8
1 year	1.079	43,6	2.173	45,8	2.146	41,1	2.859	44,6
2 years	624	25,2	1.331	28,1	1.462	28	1.532	24
3 years	229	9,3	497	10,5	708	13,5	704	11
4 years	99	4	205	4,3	286	5,5	396	6,1
Greater or Equals 5 years	152	6,1	325	6,8	394	7,5	600	9,3
Without information	174	7	5	0,1	18	0,3	3	0,04
Total	2.470	100	4.738	100	5.221	100	6.407	100

Source: SISCOLO, 2015.

In 2014, 4.8% of cytopathological tests were carried out in the same year. Considering that in the same year, the percentage of positive tests was 2% and the percentage of unsatisfactory samples was 0.6%, this adds up to 2.6%, a percentage that justifies the need for new tests in this period. This shows a high percentage of repeat Pap tests that are not necessary (INCA, 2014b).

In addition, the results regarding the periodicity of the examination suggest unnecessary repetitions, since only 11% underwent the examination within the period recommended by the Brazilian Guidelines for Cervical Cancer Screening, which recommend that after two normal annual cytological examinations, examinations should only be carried out every three years (INCA, 2011).

Reflecting the need to strengthen actions to actively seek out women for Pap smears, in accordance with the Ministry of Health's norms and guidelines. Since the result shows the high number of unnecessary repeat examinations in the same group of women, it presupposes shortcomings in screening behaviour by health professionals.

Analysing the percentage of cytopathological tests with altered results, it can be seen that there was an increase in the positivity of the tests over the years studied, ranging from 1.2% in 2011 to 2.5% in 2014 (Figure 1).

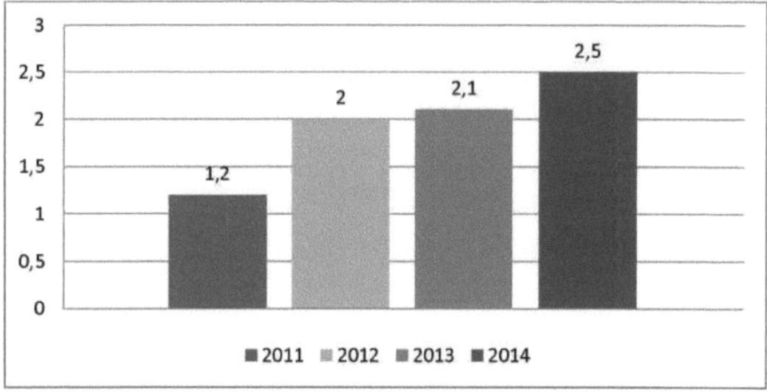

Figure 1: Positivity rate of cytopathological tests in the 16ª Health Region of Ceará-Camocim, 2011 to 2014.

Source: SISCOLO, 2015.

The results show that although there has been an increase in PI in the years evaluated, the percentage is still below the parameter recommended by the QualiCito Ordinance (Ordinance No. 3,388/2013), which is up to 3 per cent, the minimum acceptable value (BRASIL, 2013b).

With regard to the types of alteration in the cytopathological examination in the 16ª Health Region, it can be analysed that Atypia of Undetermined Significance in Squamous Cells (ASC) were the most frequent variations, with rates above 70%; followed by Low Grade Intraepithelial Lesions (LSIL) with an average percentage of

9.58%. Evaluating the percentage of tests with a diagnosis of High Grade Intraepithelial Lesion (HSIL), it can be seen that the result found corresponds to an average of 0.25%, which is below the recommended value, which is greater than or equal to 0.4% (Table 4).

Table 4: Type of alteration in the cytopathological test in women aged 25 to 64 in the 16ª health region of Ceará-Camocim, 2011 to 2014.

Changes	2011		2012		2013		2014	
	N	%	N	%	N	%	N	%
Atypia of significance	5 3	70,6	200	84	244	88,4	386	86,1
undetermined Injury	1 1	14,8	23	9,6	20	7,2	30	6,7
low-grade intraepithelial lesion	9	12	11	4,8	11	4,6	29	6,4
High-grade intraepithelial carcinoma	2	2,6	4	1,6	1	0,3	3	0,6
invader Adenocarcinomas	0	0,0	0	0,0	0	0	0	0,0
Total	7 5	100	238	100	276	100	448	100

Source: SISCOLO, 2015.

The proportion of ASCs, since it is characterised as an inconclusive result, should not represent 60% or more of the altered results; since this result portrays a diagnosis of uncertainty, necessitating the request for a new test, as well as monitoring the case (INCA, 2011). Furthermore, this result is not a definitive diagnosis, as this category does not represent a biological entity, but rather a mixture of differential diagnoses and diagnostic difficulties (INCA, 2014b).

High percentages of CSAs suggest problems in the sample, in the laboratory analysis or in both phases, as this indicator indirectly measures the quality of these stages, but does not make it possible to assess the quality of the process in isolation. In this context, it is expected that 4 or 5 per cent of all tests will be classified as ASC, as values above this percentage require evaluation and indicate a need for training among laboratory professionals (BORTOLON et al., 2012).

Analysing the proportion of tests with a diagnosis of High Grade Intraepithelial Lesion (HSIL) among the cytopathological tests carried out in the period studied, it can be seen that the result of 0.02% is far below the figure for the previous year.

of the established standard of greater than or equal to 0.4 per cent, when assessing this proportion (INCA, 2014b).

Considering that the detection of this type of lesion is the main objective of cervical cancer screening programmes, it can be inferred that in order to achieve the main objective of screening, there needs to be greater investment in the implementation of quality control for providers, as well as greater qualification for the professionals involved in collecting the material to be examined. Since it is through the correct identification of the type of alteration, together with diagnostic confirmation, treatment and appropriate follow-up, that the evolution of the lesion into cancer can be avoided, reducing its incidence and mortality.

CONCLUSION

This study made it possible to understand and describe cervical cancer screening in the 16ª Health Region of Ceará/ Camocim between 2011 and 2014.

In general, the findings show that there has been an annual increase in the number of cytological examinations carried out in the region studied, but it is not possible to say whether there has been an increase in the number of women examined, since the result only shows the number of examinations carried out and although the municipality did not reach the target for the ratio of cervical cytopathological examinations in target women, the figures found in the study show positive variations in the supply of preventive examinations in the region.

It was also concluded that unnecessary diagnostic and therapeutic procedures were characteristic of this study, increasing the cost of healthcare, as well as the presence of high percentages of atypia of undetermined significance, thus demonstrating the need for well-established protocols and the urgent need for continuing education for primary care professionals so that these diagnoses are of good quality.

One of the limitations in carrying out the study was the significant number of blank/unknown entries regarding women's schooling and race/colour, corresponding to 98% of the data in the period assessed. The aim of this study was to assess sociodemographic information in order to draw up a profile of this population; however, the significant absence of this data prevented the investigation of these variables.

The research also points to shortcomings in the early detection of lesions in the municipalities in the region. This is because tests were carried out on women outside the priority age group and a high number of cytologies were collected in periods that were not recommended. This reflects the need for studies to assess the strategies adopted by primary health care teams to attract women to undergo cytopathological examinations for cervical cancer screening.

Initiatives aimed at alerting women and the community in general to the importance of cervical cancer prevention make it possible to seek out the female population that is not participating in health services. Analyses are also needed to recognise who these women are and the factors associated with not having a Pap test.

In addition, the results and discussions of the study could help managers and health professionals to plan actions that strengthen the prevention and control of cervical cancer and, at the same time, improve women's health care. It is worth noting that, in terms of health management and planning, carrying out screening actions in accordance with the recommended guidelines optimises spending and reduces cervical cancer morbidity and mortality.

REFERENCES

BORGES MFSO, DOTTO LMG, KOIFMAN RJ, CUNHA MA, MUNIZ PT. Prevalence of cervical cancer screening in Rio Branco,

Acre, Brazil, and factors associated with not having the test. **Cadernos de Saúde Pública,** v.28, n.6, p.1156-1166, 2012.

BORTOLON PC, SILVA MAF, CORRÊA FM, DIAS MBK, KNUPP VMAO, ASSIS M, et al. Evaluation of the Quality of Cervical Cytopathology Laboratories in Brazil. **Revista Brasileira de Cancerologia**, v.58, n.3, p.435- 444, 2012.

BRAZIL. Brazilian Institute of Geography and Statistics. Cities. 2010a.

BRAZIL. Ministry of Health. Health Care Secretariat. Primary Care Department. Screening / Ministry of Health, Secretariat of Health Care, Department of Primary Care. - Brasília: Ministry of Health, 2010b.

BRAZIL. Ministry of Health. Control of cervical and breast cancers. 2.ed. Brasília (DF): Ministry of Health, 2013a. Standards and Technical Manuals).

BRAZIL. Ordinance No. 3388 of 30 December 2013. Redefines the National Qualification in Cytopathology in the prevention of cervical cancer (QualiCito), within the scope of the Health Care Network for People with Chronic Diseases. Brasília (DF): Ministry of Health; 2013b.

BRAZIL. Early Detection Newsletter. Bulletin year 6, n.2. Brasilia (DF): Ministry of Health, 2015.

CARDOSO CL, SANTOS EF, FRANÇA AMB, CAVALCANTE TCS, LIMA KBM. Analysis of the coverage of cytopathological tests in the state of Alagoas. **Caderno de Graduação-Ciências Biológicas e da Saúde-UNIT/AL**, v.2, n.2, p.31-42, 2014.

CEARÁ. State Health Secretariat. Review of the Master Plan for the Regionalisation of Health Actions and Services-PDR of the State of Ceará 2014.

DERCHAIN S, TEIXEIRA JC, ZEFERINO LC. Organized, Population-based Cervical Cancer Screening Program: It Would Be a Good Time for Brazil Now. **Brazilian Journal of Gynaecology and Obstetrics**, v.38, n.4, p.161-163, 2016.

DIAS MBK; GLAUCIA J; ASSIS TM. Cervical cancer screening in Brazil: analysing Siscolo data from 2002 to 2006. **Epidemiologia e Serviços de Saúde**, v.19, n.3, p.293-306, 2010.

INCA. National Cancer Institute. Brazilian guidelines for cervical cancer screening. Rio de Janeiro (RJ): INCA, 2011.

INCA. National Cancer Institute. Estimate 2014: Cancer Incidence in Brazil. Rio de Janeiro (RJ): INCA, 2014a.

INCA. National Cancer Institute. Cervical cancer control action indicator datasheet. Rio de Janeiro (RJ): INCA, 2014b.

INCA. José Alencar Gomes da Silva National Cancer Institute. Coordination of Prevention and Surveillance 2016 estimate: cancer incidence in Brazil / José Alencar Gomes da Silva National Cancer Institute - Rio de Janeiro: INCA, 2015a.

INCA. National Cancer Institute. Evaluation of indicators for early detection of cervical and breast cancers - Brazil and regions, 2013. Rio de Janeiro (RJ): INCA, 2015b.

KUSCHNIR R. Facing cervical cancer. In: KUSCHNIR R, FAUSTO MCR organisers. Management of Healthcare Networks. Rio de Janeiro (RJ): Fiocruz; 2014. p.19-34.

NAVARRO C, FONSECA AJ, SIBAJEV A, SOUZA CIA, ARAÚJO DS, TELES DAF et al . Cervical cancer screening coverage in a high incidence region. **Revista de Saúde Pública**, v.49, p.17, 2015.

SILVA DSM, SILVA AMN, BRITO LMO, GOMES SRL, NASCIMENTO MDSB, CHEIN MBC. Cervical cancer screening in the state of Maranhão, Brazil. **Ciências e Saúde Coletiva**, v.19, n.4, p.1163-1170, 2014.

SILVEIRA RS, SILVA AMP, ARAÚJO AC, TORRES TB, ALBUQUERQUE IMN, BRITO MCC. A preventive approach to cervical cancer with women of childbearing age. **SANARE** (Sobral, Online), v.14, n.1, p.58-64, 2015.

THULER LCS; BERGMANN A; CASADO L. Profile of patients with cervical cancer in Brazil, 2000-2009: A Secondary Study. **Revista Brasileira de Cancerologia**, v.58, n.3, p.351-7, 2012.

WHO. World Health Organisation. Comprehensive cervical cancer prevention and control: a healthier future for girls and women. Geneva: World Health Organisation; 2013.

WHO. World Health Organisation. Comprehensive Cervical Cancer Control: A Guide to Essential Practice. 2nd edition. Geneva: World Health Organisation; 2014.

CHAPTER 10

HEALTH CARE PROVIDED BY THE FAMILY HEALTH STRATEGY TEAM IN CAJAZEIRAS, PARAÍBA: AN ANALYSIS OF USERS' PERCEPTIONS

Maria José Alves Anacleto
Maura Vanessa Silva Sobreira
Wenya Sarmento Sobrinho
Weslley Epifanio Sarmento
Francisco Regis da Silva
Francisco José Maia Pinto

INTRODUCTION

An essential pillar in the construction of the new primary care model is humanisation, which, according to the proposal of the Family Health Strategy (ESF), aims to contemplate it by establishing a bond between professionals/users/families, through the team taking responsibility for resolving the community's health problems (SILVEIRA et al., 2004).

Welcoming in the health field has been associated with an action, a space or a place, with a comfortable environment, with reception and administrative triage proposing the referral of interventions. All of these are fundamental, but when taken in isolation and on a one-off basis they miss the point. Therefore, welcoming goes beyond this, as it is an ethical and professional attitude (ABBÊS; MASSARO, 2004).

However, the notion of welcoming has been limited to a professional attitude of kindness and favour; or even translates into administrative reception, a comfortable environment and triage action. However, welcoming is understood as the adoption of a posture of closeness and accountability during the development of care and management actions, favouring trust and commitment between users, teams and services (BRASIL, 2004).

Thus, welcoming is more than just qualified screening or interested listening; it presupposes a set of activities consisting of listening, problem identification and problem-solving interventions, expanding the health team's capacity to respond, reducing the centralisation of medical consultations and making better use of the potential of other professionals (TEIXEIRA; SOLLA, 2006).

Thus, according to Merhy et al. (1997), **"Welcoming and bonding depend on the way health work is produced".** Welcoming makes it possible to regulate access by offering more appropriate actions and services, contributing to user satisfaction. The bond between professional and user encourages autonomy and citizenship, promoting user participation during service provision (CAMPOS, 2006).

It is well known that the bond with health service users increases the effectiveness of health actions and favours user participation during service provision. This space must be used to build autonomous individuals, both professionals and users, because there is no bond without the user being recognised as an individual who speaks, judges and desires, putting social control into practice (CAMPOS, 2006).

The limited perception that welcoming is merely a process of screening cases and selecting the most serious ones for emergency care can be characterised as one of the main obstacles to the implementation of this technology in health services, making it even more difficult for the population to accept it, which justifies studies aimed at analysing, from the user's point of view, how welcoming is being developed in different realities (GUEDES; HENRIQUES; LIMA, 2013).

The service's view of welcoming was distorted by old concepts such as sorting, selection and queue organisation, something that should be better worked on by the professionals who still carry out these actions in isolation, which disfigures the real function of welcoming as a new way of organising demands in health services (GUEDES; HENRIQUES; LIMA, 2013).

Welcoming, therefore, is a techno-assistance action that presupposes a change in the professional/user relationship and their social network through technical, ethical, humanitarian and solidarity parameters, recognising the user as a subject and active participant in the health production process (BRASIL, 2004).

Reception, in its different configurations, stands out as a process under construction in the Unified Health System (SUS), which must be able to include users in services and, at the same time, empower health professionals and managers to build democratic, ethical and reflective spaces for the construction of a new care model, capable of producing subjects, care and health (MITRE; ANDRADE; COTTA, 2012).

Thus, by expanding users' access to the SUS in Primary Health Care (PHC), when associated with the presence of professionals trained to listen actively to their demands, it enables autonomy, citizenship and co-responsibility in the production of health care. In addition, it can effectively contribute to overcoming the myth, built up over the years, that the health care provided by public services is of poor quality and its professionals unqualified, and that the best services are in the private sector (MITRE; ANDRADE; COTTA, 2012).

Access and reception are essential elements of care in order to have an effective impact on the state of health of the individual and the community. There have been numerous problems with access and reception in basic health services. There are services with physical areas so small that they don't even have a waiting room, others which, even though they have a good place to wait, haven't found measures to extinguish the queues. There are still others where, due to the high level of pent-up demand, there is commercialisation of places in the queue. Sometimes the material conditions are good and they try to provide good service, but the reception staff are not properly qualified or, on the contrary, a good reception, screening and pre-consultation service is set up which culminates in poor service at the time of the consultation, in which cold, dehumanised and disinterested relationships are established (RAMOS, 2003).

Faced with the reality of Brazil's public Family Health Units (USF), the National Humanisation Policy (PNH) aimed to expand access and reduce queues and waiting times by proposing reception with risk classification as a potentially decisive intervention in reorganising the flow of care in the network and implementing health promotion. This policy aims to extrapolate the local management space to assert itself in everyday health practices, in the coexistence of macro and micro policies (BRASIL, 2004).

The SUS guidelines point to resoluteness as one of the main challenges to be faced in consolidating the system and promoting the population's health. However, resolutiveness has sometimes been offered from a complaint-conduct perspective, as is often seen in the care offered by overcrowded USFs (DAL PAI; LAUTERT, 2011).

Thus, the interest in developing this research on welcoming arose from an experience in a Family Health Strategy (ESF) during the supervised internship of the Undergraduate Nursing Course. It is essential that the user is welcomed, from the reception to the care provided by the service professional.

Studies on welcoming have become increasingly relevant, given that welcoming positively influences the health of the population in the area. Therefore, this research could serve as a source of knowledge about the importance of the user being well assisted, the protagonist of health care, with the aim of awakening professionals to develop strategies and ethical attitudes that reduce the damage caused by dehumanised relationships and thus improve the quality of life of users and make the Unified Health System (SUS) a policy that works.

With this in mind, the aim of this study was to investigate users' perceptions of reception and to identify favourable and unfavourable conditions in the reception of users by the Family Health Strategy Team in Cajazeiras, Paraíba, Brazil.

METHODS

In order to meet the objectives presented, an exploratory field study was carried out with a quantitative approach. Field research was used in order to obtain information and/or knowledge about a problem for which an answer is sought, or a hypothesis that is to be proved and to discover new phenomena and/or the relationships between them (MARCONI; LAKATOS, 2002).

The study site was a Family Health Unit in the Sol Nascente neighbourhood in the municipality of Cajazeiras, Paraíba, Brazil. The city of Cajazeiras is located in the hinterland of the state, 463 km from the capital João Pessoa, and has a territorial extension of 566 km^2 according to data from the Brazilian Institute of Geography and Statistics (IBGE) (IBGE, 2010). Only one health unit was chosen as the study site because, at the time of the research, it was the only one working with reception.

The population was made up of 1,270 families, which corresponds to 4,000 people registered at the Health Unit. The sample was non-probabilistic and intentional, corresponding to 5% of the population, i.e. 200 users registered with the ESF. The inclusion criteria were: the user must be over 18 years old, have been registered at the unit for at least 1 year and agree to take part in the study and sign the Informed Consent Form (ICF) at the time of data collection.

The data was collected after the research project was approved by the Research Ethics Committee of Faculdade Santa Maria (FSM/Paraíba), CAAE 05571812.8.0000.5180, substantiated opinion number 168.879. Thus, all the prerogatives contained in Resolution 466/2012 were complied with (BRASIL, 2012).

A structured questionnaire containing objective questions with more than one alternative was used to collect the data. Data was collected at the ESF when users were at the reception desk. The data was analysed using descriptive statistics with simple and relative frequencies using Microsoft Excel®, 2010. They were then presented in tables and graphs and discussed in accordance with the literature pertinent to the proposed study.

All the participants signed the Free and Informed Consent Form (FICF), which proves that all the subjects' rights were guaranteed, in terms of their voluntary participation, data confidentiality, anonymity and freedom to refuse to participate or withdraw their consent at any stage of the research. The participants received clarification on the objectives and methods of the research, through the information contained in the (ICF), which was duly signed.

RESULTS

The data was categorised in two stages. The first contains data related to the sociodemographic characterisation of the sample, and the second contains data related to the research objective.

Characterisation of the participants

Firstly, the participants in the survey were characterised in terms of gender, marital status, schooling, age group, monthly income and length of time registered at the Basic Health Unit (Table 01).

Table 03. Characterisation of users according to gender, marital status, schooling, age group, monthly income and length of registration. Cajazeiras - PB, 2012.

VARIABLES	N°	%
SEX		
Female	150	75,0
Male	50	25,0
CIVIL STATUS		
Single	60	30,0
Married	111	55,5
Widowed	12	6,0
Divorced	13	6,5
Others	4	2,0
SCHOOLING		
Illiterate	8	4,0
Primary Education Complete	18	9,0
Elementary School Incomplete	98	49,0
Completed high school	57	28,5
Secondary school incomplete	8	4,0
Higher education completed	3	1,5
Higher education incomplete	8	4,0
AGE GROUP		
18 to 30 years old	70	35,0
31 to 40 years old	44	22,0
41 to 50 years old	41	20,5
51 to 60 years old	26	13,0

61 to 80 years old	19	9,5
MONTHLY INCOME		
Minus 1 salary	108	54,0
1 to 3 salaries	89	44,5
3 to 6 salaries	1	0,5
6 to 8 salaries	2	1,0
REGISTRATION TIME/YEARS		
1 a 2	57	28,5
2 a 4	96	48,0
4 a 6	42	21,0
6 a 8	5	2,5

Source: Research data, 2012.

Table 01 shows that the prevalent age of the participants was 18 to 30 (35%), followed by 31 to 40 (22%), 41 to 50 (20.5%), 51 to 60 (13%) and 61 to 80 (9.5%). There were also more females than males (75 per cent) (25 per cent). With regard to marital status, 30% of users were single, 55.5% married, 6% widowed, 6.5% divorced and 2% other. With regard to monthly income, the majority of users earned less than the minimum wage (54%).

With regard to schooling, 49 per cent of those interviewed had incomplete primary education.

With regard to the length of time users had been registered, 48.4 per cent had been registered for between 2 and 4 years, which shows that users have been linked to the ESF for only a short time.

Reception and favourable and unfavourable conditions

With regard to understanding reception, Graph 01 shows the main perceptions highlighted by the study participants.

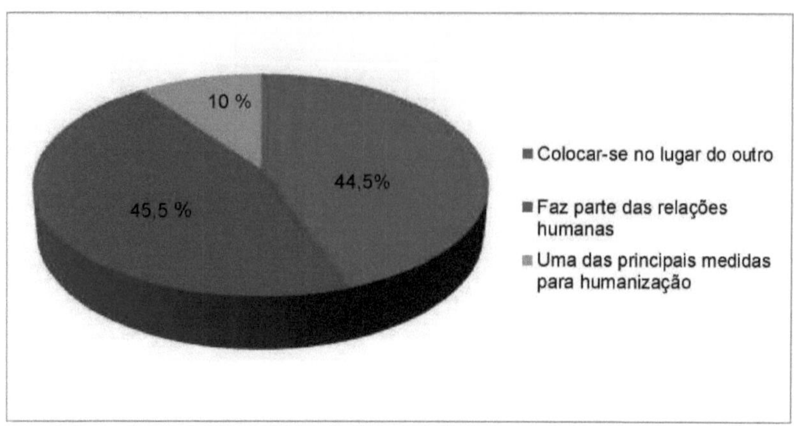

Graph 01: Users' understanding of reception. Cajazeiras - PB, 2012.

Source: Research data, 2012.

Graph 01 shows that the users' greatest understanding of welcoming in the study was that it is part of human relations (45.5%), followed by other alternatives such as putting oneself in the other person's shoes (44.5%), and one of the main actions for humanisation is welcoming (10%).

Graph 02 shows how the reception at the ESF is rated, with 5.5 per cent of users considering it excellent, 7.5 per cent very good, 17.5 per cent bad, 22.5 per cent fair and 47.50 per cent good.

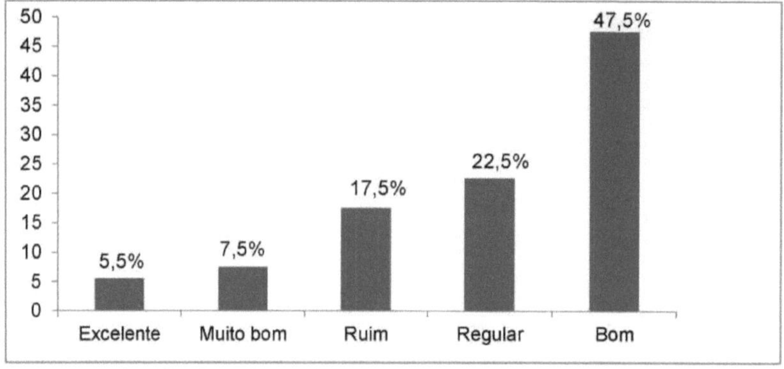

Graph 02: Classification of reception by users at the USF. Cajazeiras - PB, 2012.

Source: Research data, 2012.

Graph 03 highlights users' opinions on what contributes to welcoming people in a health centre. They stated: compliance with the professionals' timetable (22.5%), waiting time (11.5%), quality of care (45.5%), qualification of health professionals (20.5%).

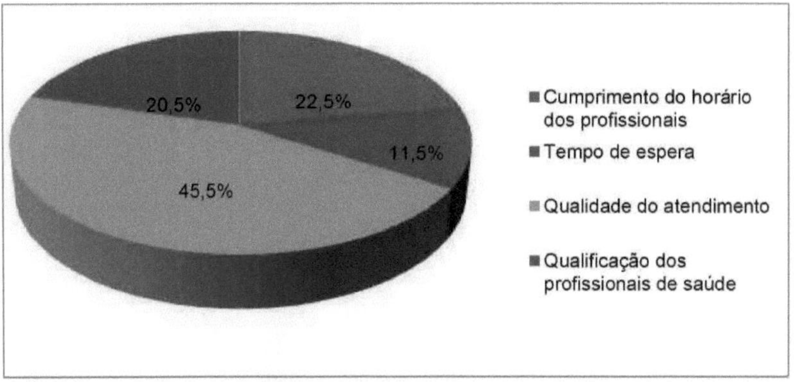

Graph 03: Contributions of reception to the health unit, according to users. Cajazeiras - PB, 2012.

Source: Research data, 2012.

Graph 04 describes the difficulties identified in the reception provided by the ESF, according to users.

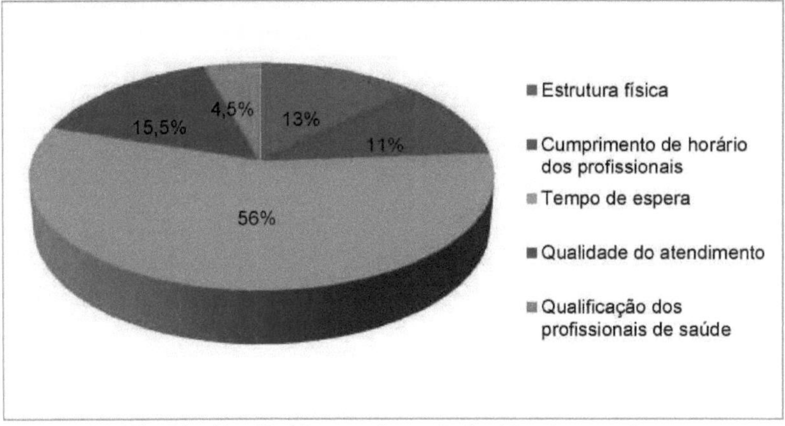

Graph 04: Difficulties identified in reception at the health unit, according to users. Cajazeiras - PB, 2012.

Source: Research data, 2012.

Analysing the difficulties related to the process and organisation of the ESF, it was found that users perceive that the unfavourable conditions are related to the inadequate physical area, excessive demand and the lack of a doctor in the unit. Of the users who took part in the survey, (4.5%) said that what hinders reception are the qualifications of the health professionals, compliance with the professionals' timetable (11%), quality of care (15.5%) and waiting times (56%).

Graph 05 shows the following factors that could be improved in the reception service: health professionals (7.5%), waiting times (21%), physical structure (21.5%), speed of booking (49%) and publicising services (1%).

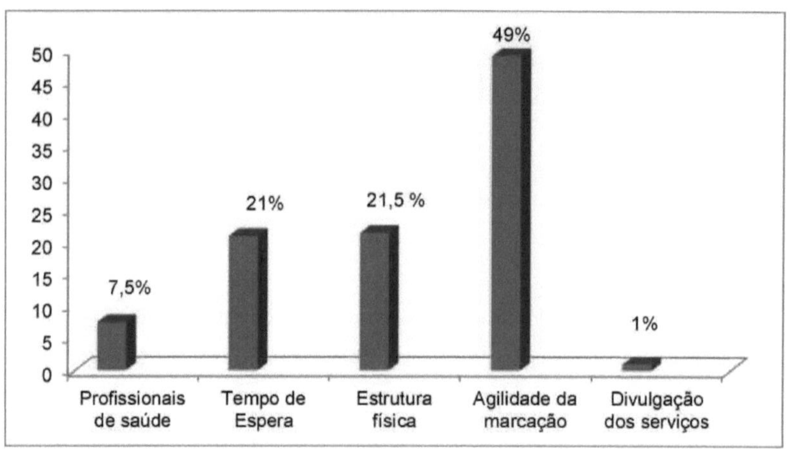

Graph 05: Suggestions for improvements in the reception provided by the ESF. Cajazeiras - PB, 2012.

Source: Research data, 2012.

DISCUSSION

Characterisation of the participants

The low educational level of the subjects surveyed (users) leads us to reflect on the difficulty that low schooling causes in the care offered by the health team. Many users have difficulty understanding and even lack information about their rights and basic actions, such as administering the medicines they use on a daily basis.

Unfortunately, in today's society, few people have access to a decent salary and housing. As a result, the lack of leisure time is present in the daily lives of these families and these are factors that contribute to the population becoming ill, causing them to seek out curative health services more often.

Registering the population living in the territory is essential, as the Family Health Strategy team is responsible for health surveillance actions that go beyond using the Basic Health Unit for health care. In addition, the production of information on the population's health requires knowledge of the total number of residents in the area (BRASIL, 2014).

In order for nurses, doctors and/or any other health professional to be in a position to provide comprehensive care to the population, they need to keep up to date. This highlights the fundamental role of service institutions in the ongoing development of professionals' skills, contributing to their social well-being and personal and professional growth, and helping to organise the work process through stages that can problematise reality and produce change.

Thus, for Santos (2002), it is in everyday life, in the concrete space of the family, that the system's professionals, in interaction with the family, seek to build health, prioritising protection, the promotion of self-care and the exchange of solidarity, thus seeking to move away from the dependent biomedical model, centred on the disease. We can see that the philosophy behind it is more than a simple extension of services, as it encourages a practice that favours criticism, change and the construction of knowledge.

These findings lead us to reflect that welcoming needs to be considered a work tool that incorporates human relations, appropriate for all health professionals, in all sectors, in every sequence of acts and modes that make up the work process, not limited to the act of receiving (FRACOLLI; BERTOLOZZI, 2009).

Pinheiro (2009) points out that the challenge of humanisation is to create a new culture of care, based on the centrality of the subjects in the collective construction of the SUS. For this proposal to be consolidated, workers need to be motivated, with decent working conditions and compatible salaries. Care protocols and work routines must be drawn up, and investment must be made in continuing education for the teams, in order to rethink the health care model and constantly assess the difficulties that arise in the collective health work process. Users' participation in this process is therefore of the utmost importance.

Reception and favourable and unfavourable conditions

In this context, it can be seen that welcoming is not just seen as a measure of humanisation, it goes further, being perceived as something intrinsic to being human, of being present in the various social relationships.

According to Fracolli and Bertolozzi (2009), reception in health services has been considered a process specifically of human relations, as it must be carried out by all health workers and in all sectors of care. It is not limited to the act of receiving, but constitutes a sequence of acts and modes that make up the health work process. It is one of the main actions for humanising care. Access and welcoming are therefore essential elements of care in order to have an effective impact on the state of health of the individual and the community

When welcoming is seen as an emergency service, triage at the door can perpetuate the exclusion of users and communities from the SUS, hindering adherence to the therapeutic project, bonding and co-responsibility (MITRE; ANDRADE; COTTA, 2012).

> As part of this policy, welcoming can be seen as a strategy for applying the guiding principles of the Unified Health System (SUS), based on qualified listening that allows the user's needs, risks and vulnerabilities to be identified, in order to offer the appropriate referral for these needs, according to these principles. But the different definitions of welcoming converge around communication, being considered a way of listening in which empathy is established, showing interest in the other person's speech (PINHEIRO, 2009).
>
> In this way, Merhy et al. (1997) include welcoming as an initial element of the health work process, centred on soft technologies, which refer to care in its broadest sense, not requiring specific professional knowledge in each area. This differs from the current organisation of health services, which is centred on hard technologies, intrinsically dependent on equipment, and on soft technologies, characterised by the mastery of a specific core of knowledge, such as medical or nursing consultations.
>
> The need to improve reception arises when neglect in the health area is present, as well as arrogance, lack of interest in providing qualified care and the commercialism present in many professions. In this sense, to humanise is also to invest in improving the working conditions of healthcare professionals, and to achieve

benefits for the health and quality of life of all those involved in this process.

Therefore, it is clear that the participants in the survey like to be attended to by professionals who provide a proper welcome, with dialogue and the creation of a bond, culminating in a return to routine appointments at the UBS, which is beneficial for the subjects, even as a way of reducing suffering.

These complaints about the organisational aspect refer to what is still insufficient, precarious or non-existent. It is clear that if there is to be a significant change in the care model and in the process of humanising care, it is necessary to redirect the organisation and distribution of actions and services in such a way as to respond satisfactorily to demands, as well as to health needs, and in order to do this, it is necessary to associate practices of attending to spontaneous demand and health surveillance (SILVEIRA, et al., 2004).

It's clear that all the participants in the research came to the unit to have their needs met. This is **a "moment of saying" in** which the user and the professional present themselves with the marks of their lives and where words and gestures are part of a complex communication. Capturing the unique health needs at this moment requires the professional to be open to leaning towards the user, to listening, to establishing bonds of trust. It implies welcoming the other, offering space for speech and dialogue (BRASIL, 2004).

Thus, for Silveira et al. (2004) an essential pillar in the construction of the new primary care model is humanisation, and the ESF aims to contemplate this proposal by establishing a bond between professionals/users/families, through the responsibility of the health team and the community.

It is worth emphasising that in their speeches, users spoke of the importance of qualifying the worker-subject relationship, in order to attend to all the people who seek health services, guaranteeing universal accessibility and welcoming them, listening, giving a positive response, being able to solve individuals' health problems.

At the initial moment of reception, without the intention of establishing any therapeutic interventions, emergency consultations, medical referrals to specialists and/or the scheduling of appointments at the unit itself would be generated. The main objective is to listen to the user and identify their needs, in order to offer them the most appropriate care possibilities according to their demands. The aim is to prevent people from failing to attend appointments (RAMOS, 2003).

Therefore, according to Santos (2002) who corroborates Scholze (2006), welcoming attitudes and actions based on qualified listening by all health workers, guided by the concepts of field and nucleus, competence and co-responsibility, would give health professionals and teams greater autonomy. In this way, the subjects, workers and users would benefit and, consequently, quality of life would be produced, the main objective of the welcoming system, implying a transformation in the way the population has been given access from the "front door", as well as changes in the actions that result from this first contact, such as scheduling appointments and programming services. Thus, as well as contributing to humanisation and improving the quality of care, it is a strategy for reorienting professional practices and their relationships with users in order to improve their well-being.

CONCLUSION

Welcoming means the worker's attitude of putting themselves in the user's shoes to feel out what their needs are and, as far as possible, meeting them or directing them to the point in the system that is capable of responding to those demands. It's more than just receiving or sorting, it's going beyond, being attentive, seeking in a humanised way to provide care and resolve issues according to professional limits and the questions that are asked.

Thus, the data collected in this study shows that reception in the PSF at the Sol Nascente Health Unit in Cajazeiras, PB, is still a culture under construction, since the programme is relatively new and presupposes a complete reorientation of the current care model.

In this sense, the culture that professionals have about welcoming is related to the following concepts: "receiving well", "listening well", "being attentive", "understanding" and "showing solidarity". These concepts corroborate the concept of welcoming in the context of health services and are so emphasised in the literature.

In this way, the humanisation of care is perceived by professionals as a holistic way of caring, seeing the user as an individual with fragilities. It's a moment that brings the user and the professional closer together, recognising the user's needs and identifying priorities in care. Humanisation is seen, however, as an opportunity to provide guidance to the user, qualifying care. Therefore, humanisation also involves resolutive care.

Therefore, despite the institutional, professional and social limitations reported, these professionals experience the practice of welcoming on a daily basis, extrapolating even their professional training, which generally qualifies them for curative actions.

REFERENCES

ABBÊS, C.; MASSARO, A. **Acolhimento com Avaliação e Classificação de Risco: Um Paradigma Ético-Estético no fazer em Saúde**. Brasília: Ministry of Health 2004, 49p. Available at:<http://www.slab.uff.br/textos/texto84.pdf>. Accessed on: 28 July 2016.

BRAZIL. Ministry of Health. Executive Secretariat. Technical Centre for the National Humanisation Policy. **HumanizaSUS: reception with risk assessment and classification: an ethical-aesthetic paradigm in healthcare**. Ministry of Health. Brasília: 2004. Available at: <http://bvsms.saude.gov.br/bvs/publicacoes/acolhimento.pdf>. Accessed on: 28 July 2016.

BRAZIL. Ministry of Health. National Health Council. National Research Ethics Committee. Norms for research involving human beings (CNS Resolution 466/12). Brasília: 2012.

BRAZIL. National Council of Health Secretaries. **Primary Care and Health Promotion**. National Council of Health Secretaries. Brasília: CONASS, 2007.

CAMPOS, G.W.S. **Paradoxical effects of the decentralisation of the Unified Health System in Brazil**. In: FLEURY, S. (Org.) Democracy, decentralisation and development: Brazil and Spain. Editora FGV, 2006.

DAL PAI, D.; LAUTERT, L. Suffering in nursing work: reflexes of the "empty discourse" in the reception with risk classification. **Esc. Anna Nery**, v. 15, n. 3, p. 524-530, 2011.

FRACOLLI, L. A.; BERTOLOZZI, M.R. A **abordagem do processo saúde-doença das famílias e do coletivo.** Nursing manual. Rio de Janeiro, 2003.

GUEDES, M.V.C.; HENRIQUES, A.C.P.T.; LIMA, M.M.N. Acolhimento em um serviço de emergência: percepção dos usuários. **Revista Brasileira de Enfermagem**, v.66, n.1, p.31-37, 2013.

IBGE. **Brazilian Institute of Geography and Statistics.** Population Census 2010. Available at: <http://www.ibge.gov.br/cidadesat/painel/painel.php?codmun=250370>. Accessed on 12 May 2016.

MARCONI, M.A; LAKATOS, E.M. **Técnicas de pesquisa**. São Paulo: Atlas, 2002.

MERHY, E.E.; et al. In search of tools to analyse health technologies: information and the day-to-day life of a service, questioning and managing health work. In: Merhy E.E.O.R. (Organisers). **Acting in health:** a challenge for the public. São Paulo: Editora Hucitec, 1997. p.113-50.

MITRE, S.M.; ANDRADE, E.I.G.; COTTA, R.M.M. Avanços e desafios do acolhimento na operationalização e qualificação do Sistema Único de Saúde na Atenção Primária: um resgate da produção bibliográfica do Brasil. **Ciências e Saúde Coletiva**, v.17, n.8, p.2071-208, 2012.

PINHEIRO, N.O.; et al. Grupo de Trabalho Serviço Social na Saúde. **Parâmetros para a Atuação de Assistentes Sociais na Saúde (Preliminary Version)**. Brasilia, 2009.

RAMOS, D.D. Acesso e acolhimento aos usuários em uma unidade de saúde de Porto Alegre, Rio Grande do Sul. **Cadernos de Saúde Pública**, v.19, n.1, p.27-34, 2003.

SANTOS, B.R.L.; et al. Formando o enfermeiro para o cuidado à saúde da família: um olhar sobre o ensino de graduação. **Revista Brasileira de Enfermagem**, v.53, special edition, p.49-59, 2002.

TEIXEIRA, C.F.; SOLLA, J.P. **Modelo de atenção à saúde**: vigilância e saúde da família. Salvador: Editora EDUFBA, 2006. 237p.

SILVEIRA, M.F.A.; et al. Acolhimento no Programa Saúde da Família: um caminho para humanização da atenção à saúde. **Cogitare Enfermagem**, v.9, n.1, p.71-78, 2004.

SCHOLZE, A.S.; et al. The implementation of welcoming in the work process of family health teams. **Revista Espaço para a Saúde**, v.8, n.1, p.7- 12, 2006.

CHAPTER 11

THE IMPORTANCE OF EXCLUSIVE BREASTFEEDING IN THE DEVELOPMENT OF NEWBORN BABIES

Lorena Samilla Sales Lucas

Thamyres Fortaleza Monteiro

Mara Iza Holanda de Almeida

Rafaella Maria Monteiro Sampaio

INTRODUCTION

Breastfeeding is when a child receives breast milk, either directly from the breast or milked, regardless of whether they are receiving any other food or liquid, including non-human milk. Breast milk is a fluid secreted and produced by the mammary glands to meet nutritional, defensive and physiological needs, providing all the nutrients, minerals and vitamins necessary for the growth of the newborn. Because it has a protective effect, it is so important during the first six months of life, when exclusive breastfeeding is recommended, due to its beneficial effect on the survival of these children (FOX, 2008).

Human milk is a food produced through a normal physiological process that is standard for our species. The distinct characteristics observed in relation to other milks are of a quantitative and qualitative nature, since it is biologically adapted to the characteristics and needs of infants, and gradually changes its quantity and composition constantly due to the interaction between mother and child. In the first few days of a neonate's life, human milk is in the form of colostrum, then transitional milk and, from the second week onwards, mature milk (CORDERO, 2005).

It is well known that breastfeeding is the best and most efficient way of meeting the nutritional needs of newborn babies. Children who are exclusively breastfed are less likely to die when compared to those who receive complementary and mixed breastfeeding, i.e. those who use milk formulas (LUCAS; COLE, 1990; CAMPESTRINI, 2006). In addition to being one of the most important practices for the healthy development and growth of a newborn, human milk provides nutritional and immunological benefits due to its nutrients. It also has a protective effect against infections, obesity, respiratory diseases and other pathologies (CAMPESTRINI, 2006).

Studies have shown that children who are exclusively breastfed for the first six months of life grow faster than those who receive infant formula and/or other types of food, and even children who are weaned early are more likely to develop childhood obesity, which is caused by the high energy value of this food (WHO, 1998; KRAMER et al., 2002; NEJAR et al., 2004).

Other studies carried out in southern Brazil have shown that dietary patterns are associated with the growth of children in their first month of life, but that by the third month of life, children who were exclusively breastfed had a tendency to gain more weight compared to those who were weaned early. There was also an inversion in terms of growth. These differences occurred between three and six months, when children who had been weaned grew faster than those who were exclusively breastfed. After six months, growth was similar between the two groups of children, but weaned children tended to gain more weight, which could have a detrimental effect on the child's health, leading to childhood obesity (VICTORA et al., 1998).

Thus, this study was carried out with the aim of analysing the growth of children according to the food they receive and helping mothers with guidance, since it was identified that there was little frequency or difficult conditions in the professional's work in terms of nutritional monitoring of children. It is believed that this research will provide guidance and action on the importance of breastfeeding for children's growth, sensitising mothers to the importance of breastfeeding for their children's health and development. In view of this, the main objective of the study was to analyse the importance of exclusive breastfeeding for the development and nutritional status of newborns.

METHODS

This is a descriptive study with a quantitative approach and a cross-sectional design, in which children were assessed according to their weight and height, in order to analyse their growth and find out what influence breast milk has on this development. The study included children aged 0-6 months who were being exclusively breastfed, as well as those who were receiving other types of food.

The data was collected at health centres in the city of Trairi-CE between April and May 2016. In the study, the children were divided into groups: group 1 was made up of exclusively breastfed children and group 2 was made up of those who were already on complementary and mixed feeding. Fifty children were monitored, 25 in each group.

To collect the data, an investigative form was given to the mothers, the aim of which was to find out and obtain information about the participant's diet, which included objective questions about the period of breastfeeding and the diet they were eating. The data was collected through interviews with the participants' parents. The data was tabulated and analysed using Microsoft Excel® version 2010 spreadsheets.

The mothers signed an informed consent form authorising their children to undergo the nutritional assessment. Nutritional assessments were then carried out, using anthropometric measurements such as weight/height, weight/age, height/age and BMI/age, based on the curves used to classify these children. For this procedure, weight (kg) and height (cm) were measured using a digital scale, where the child was placed on the scale on a flat surface with as few clothes as possible and a tape measure fixed to a surface in a horizontal position, i.e. lying down, measuring the distance from the feet to the top of the head.

Once this procedure had been carried out, the children were classified according to the cut-off points adopted by the WHO (2011) and analysed using the growth and development charts in the WHO Anthro software.

The data was presented in tables and graphs, using descriptive statistics (simple and relative frequencies, means and standard deviation).

The research was carried out in accordance with the ethical principles of Resolution 466/2012, and was approved by the Ethics Committee of the Estácio do Ceará University Centre (approval number 1.523.423).

RESULTS

When the sample was analysed, it was found that of the 50 children who took part in the study, 28 (56%) were female, 11 (22%) were receiving exclusive breast milk and 17 (34%) were already on a mixed diet. As a result, the highest prevalence of children feeding only on breast milk was among boys, with 14 (28%) and 8 (16%) who were already complementary feeders.

With regard to the age at which the children were weaned early, i.e. that they started complementary feeding, 26 per cent (n=13) would have been weaned at 3 months, 14 per cent (n=7) at 4 months and 10 per cent (n=5) at 2 months of age.

With regard to the weight of the newborns, it was found that the lowest weight in the breastfed group was 5kg and the highest was 9.1kg, with an average weight of 6.86kg. As for the group of children who use complementary feeding, the lowest weight observed was 4.9kg and the highest 10.2kg, with an average weight of 7kg. As for height, it was possible to observe that the smallest height in the breastfed group was 55cm and the largest 68.5cm, with an average height of 61cm, while in the other group the smallest height was 53cm and the largest 64.5cm, with an average height of 59.5cm.

Table 1: Growth and development parameters of the nutritional status of exclusively breastfed and supplemented newborns aged 0 to 6 months. Trairi-CE/2016.

	Children exclusively breastfed up to 6 months		**Children with complemented and mixed feeding**		**Total**	
	N	**%**	**N**	**%**	**N**	**%**
Sex						
Female	11	22%	17	34%	28	56%
Male	14	28%	8	16%	22	44%
P/A						
Suitable	19	38%	5	10%	24	48%
Risk of overweight	6	12%	20	40%	26	52%
P/I						
Suitable	25	50%	25	50%	50	100%
A/I						
Suitable	25	50%	25	50%	50	100%
BMI/I						
Suitable	19	38%	5	10%	24	48%
Risk of Overweight	6	12%	20	40%	26	52%

Values expressed as means and percentages. *Classified according to the Ministry of Health's cut-off points and the food and nutrition surveillance system - SISVAN.

Regarding the growth and development of the newborns in each group in the study in question, it was observed that the children who had been exclusively breastfed had adequate growth and development parameters according to the cut-off points adopted by the Ministry of Health. However, the group represented by the newborns who had already been given complementary or mixed feeding was found to be at risk of overweight in some parameters (Table 1).

The following graphs show the difference between development and growth, in terms of the type of feeding, during the period from 0 to 6 months of age. Graph 1 shows how children develop and grow when they are fed only breast milk, and Graph 2 shows the development of children who are already on a complementary diet of solid and liquid foods in addition to breast milk.

The graph for exclusively breastfed children shows that the curve during the period from the 2nd to the 4th month has an incidence of the cut-off points, which means that it is during this interval that the children develop the most. As for children on complementary feeding, it can be seen that during the period in which the child was not weaned, it was within the appropriate parameters and that when complementary and mixed feeding was introduced, there was an increase in its weight, making it a child at risk of being overweight.

Another difference that could be observed between the groups was that exclusively breastfed newborns developed better in terms of height than weaned ones, as they tended to gain more weight (Graphs 1 and 2).

According to the questionnaire administered to parents about breastfeeding, 50 (100%) mothers are aware of the importance of breastfeeding for their child's development and 48% (n=26) have breastfed previously. An important point to note in this questionnaire is that mothers who had previously breastfed accounted for 30% (n=15) of the mothers who weaned their child early, and the total sample of this group is 50%, i.e. a high number compared to first-time mothers, who accounted for 32% (n=16) of the sample of mothers who exclusively breastfed their children.

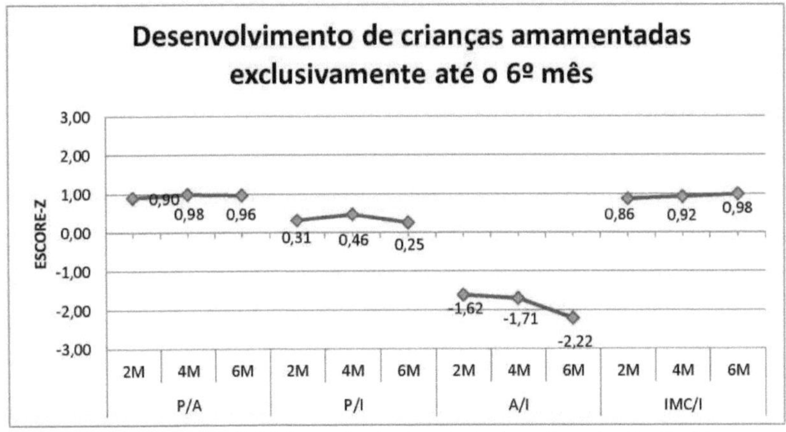

Graph 1: Development of children who feed exclusively on breast milk. Trairi-CE/2016

Values expressed as mean *Cut-off points expressed according to z-score.

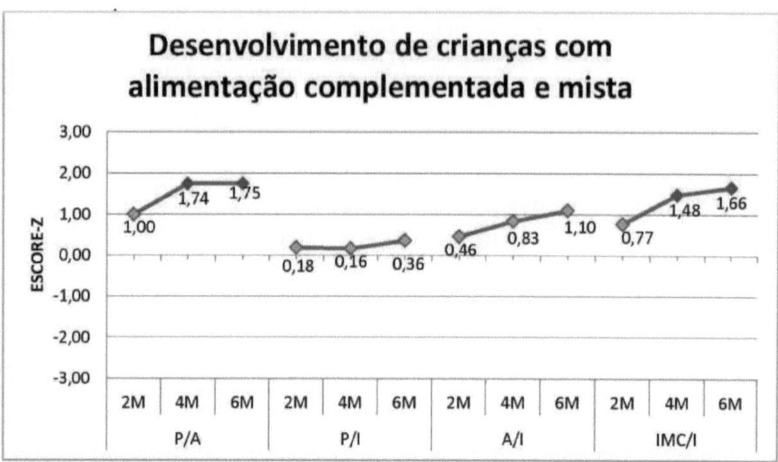

Graph 2: Development of children who eat solid and liquid foods in addition to breast milk. Trairi-CE/2016

Values expressed as mean *Cut-off points expressed according to z-score.

With regard to the ideal age to wean a child, 34% (n=17) of the mothers answered that they should wean their child at 2 years of age, 28% (n=14) when the baby no longer wants to be weaned, 22% (n=11) when the baby is 1 year old, 12% (n=6) at 6 months and 4% (n=2) did not know the answer. This question also showed that first-time mothers accounted for the largest proportion of mothers who answered 2 years (34%), which shows us that they seek more information about breastfeeding than mothers who have had other children before.

DISCUSSION

A study carried out by the National Demographic and Health Survey of Children and Women, PNDS (2006), showed that the prevalence of exclusive breastfeeding among children aged 0 to 3 months is still considered low (45 per cent), although it is higher than that found in the 1996 PNDS (40 per cent). With regard to exclusive breastfeeding in the 4 to 6 month age group, it fell to 11 per cent in 2006. It also showed that the majority of children are subject to inadequate breastfeeding practices and low quality complementary feeding. The study found that 20.5 per cent of children were fed pre-milk foods (liquids such as water, tea and other milks), 48 per cent were exclusively breastfed in the first 3 months of life; 14 per cent were already using semi-solid foods before they were 2 months old and between the 4th and 5th months of age, around a third of newborns were already completely weaned (BRASIL, 2009).

Vitolo (2008) reported that supplemented breastfeeding was 32 per cent in the 0-3 month range and 56 per cent in the 4-6 month range in 2006. 23 per cent of these children were completely weaned in the 0 to 3 month age group and 33 per cent in the 4 to 6 month age group. In the latter age group, **35 per cent of the children were already eating "salty food", which shows that** their diet is inadequate for their age (VITOLO, 2008).

According to this study, 26 per cent of the children were exclusively breastfed until they were 3 months old, 14 per cent at 4 months and 10 per cent at 2 months, and then started to eat complementary and mixed foods, such as porridge, soups, juices, teas and water.

According to the WHO, exclusive breastfeeding is recommended for 0-6 months and complementary breastfeeding until the child is 2 years old or older, as there is no advantage in starting complementary foods before 6 months of age, which could be detrimental to the baby's health. For this reason, several countries have officially adopted exclusive breastfeeding, which should be extended until the child is 6 months old (MUNIZ, 2010).

However, in developed countries, most mothers start administering other artificial foods before the 4th month and wean long before the child is 2 years old, which is the recommended age for weaning. Even though some doctors consider six months to be a prolonged period of breastfeeding and find it questionable that women breastfeed their children for more than a year (PÉREZ et al., 1994).

This study found that 34 per cent of mothers consider that the ideal age to wean their child would be at 2 years of age, 28 per cent when the baby no longer wants to, 22 per cent when the baby is 1 year old, 12 per cent at 6 months and 4 per cent didn't know how to answer. 92 per cent know how important breast milk is for their child's life, the other 8 per cent didn't know how to answer.

In 2001, the WHO published a resolution stating that babies should be exclusively breastfed for the first 6 months of their lives. This resolution was based on a study carried out in Honduras, which showed that babies fed exclusively on breast milk for 6 months grew better than babies breastfed up to the 4th month. And that supplemented feeding offered no advantage for growth, and that those exclusively breastfed for 6 months had better psychomotor development and a lower incidence of allergic and digestive manifestations (PÉREZ, 2001).

A study of preschoolers in São Paulo showed that exclusive breastfeeding for 6 months and for more than 2 years was considered a preventive factor against overweight and obesity (SIMON et al., 2009). Another study by Twells and Newhood (2012) also showed that exclusivity for 3 months was protective against obesity (TWELLS L; NEWHOOD, 2012).

Like Scott and Cobiac (2012) who said that children who are breastfed for more than 6 months are more protected from overweight and obesity in later life. Owen et al. (2005) showed that breastfeeding is largely associated with a reduced risk of developing late-onset obesity, when compared to those who received infant formula.

By analysing the data and classifying it according to the WHO cut-off points, the study showed that babies who were breastfed only would be within the appropriate growth parameters, with the highest incidence of growth between the 2nd and 4th months, settling down by the 6th month. However, babies who received complementary and mixed feeding had a higher risk of developing overweight, as they tended to gain more weight and grow less in height compared to children in the other group. In this group, it was possible to observe that there was a slight reduction in the A/I parameter from the 2nd to the 6th month

The WHO (2001) recommends that complementary feeding to breast milk, consisting of solid or liquid foods, should be introduced after 6 months of exclusive breastfeeding, as this is no longer effective in meeting the child's nutritional needs.

According to the Ministry of Health (2002), the complementary dietary pattern of children in Brazil is unfavourable, as it is introduced at an early age, in addition to the fact that taboos and beliefs contribute to the low consumption of rich foods and sources of vitamins and minerals, meaning that it does not meet their needs (BRASIL, 2002).

Overweight in the first years of life is more frequent and is related to the practice of early weaning and the spread of incorrect dietary norms, which help to develop overfeeding (CORSO et al., 2003). It is known that this is often due to the fact that some mothers, especially those from low socioeconomic backgrounds, overfeed their children out of fear that they will become malnourished, consequently leading them to become overweight (RODRIGUES, 2009).

We can therefore say that children who used exclusive breast milk up to 6 months of age had adequate, healthy and standardised growth. While those on complementary and mixed feeding only gained weight and height below what was recommended, and these children may be at greater risk of developing overweight, which is why exclusive breastfeeding in the first months of life is essential, because as we have seen, in addition to defensive and physiological actions, it also meets nutritional needs, thus providing all the nutrients and vitamins necessary for healthy growth and development.

CONCLUSION

The study showed that exclusive breastfeeding is essential in the first few months of life, because as we were shown, breast milk fully meets the nutritional, defensive and physiological needs, thus providing all the nutrients necessary for the healthy growth of newborns. It was found that children who were exclusively breastfed had better growth when compared to those who received complementary and mixed feeding, but had a greater tendency to gain weight, which could have a detrimental effect on the child's health, leading them to become overweight.

Therefore, health professionals, especially nutritionists, must support mothers and babies during the initiation and maintenance of breastfeeding, so that the practice of breastfeeding is successful. They should have a bond of trust with the mother and her family, providing information and clarifying doubts about breastfeeding and thus reinforcing its importance for the health of both the mother and the child, which, as has been shown, is essential and of great importance if the child is to develop optimally and healthily.

REFERENCES

BRAZIL. Ministry of Health. Practical guide to preparing food for children under two. Brasilia, 2002.

BRAZIL. Ministry of Health. National demographic and child and women's health survey report. Brasilia, 2009.

CAMPESTRINI S. Breastfeeding summary. Breastfeeding programme. Curitiba: Pontifical Catholic University of Paraná; 2006.

CORDERO AMJ. Composition, properties and biochemistry of human milk. Immediate principles. Madrid: Elsevier, 53-63, 2005.

CORSO ACT; BOTELHO LS; ZENI LAZR; MOREIRA EAM. Overweight in children under 6 years of age in Florianópolis. **Revista de Nutrição**, Campinas, v.16, n.1, p.21-28, 2003.

FOX PF. Milk: an overview. In: THOMPSON A; BOLAND M; SINGH H. Milk Proteins: From Expression to Food. 1. ed. London: Academic Press, 2008. p.1- 54.

KRAMER M.S.; et al. Breastfeeding and infant growth: biology or bias? **Paediatrics**. 2002.

LUCAS A; COLE TJ. Breast milk and neonatal necrotising enterocolitis. **Lancet,** 336, 1990.

MUNIZ MD. **Benefits of breastfeeding for the puerperal woman and the newborn: the role of the family health team**. Federal University of Minas Gerais, Faculty of Medicine. Formiga, 2010.

NEJAR FF; et al. Patterns of breastfeeding and energy adequacy **Caderno de Saúde Pública**, Rio de Janeiro, v. 20, n. 1, p. 37-40, 2004.

OWEN CG; RICHARD M; SMITH GD; WHINCUP PH; COOK DG. Effect of infant feeding on the risk of obesity across the life course: a quantitative review of published evidence. **Pediatrics**, Stanford, v15 n5, 2005.

PÉREZ ER; POLLITT E; LONNERDAL B; DEWEY KJ. Infant feeding policies in maternity wards and their effect on breast-feeding success: in analytical overview. **Am J. public Health**, 89 - 97, 1994.

PÉREZ ER. Development and epidemiology of child feeding indications in Ghana and Honduras: surveillance and programme evaluation applications, 2001.

RODRIGUES L. Childhood obesity. In: ACCIOLY E; SAUDERS C; LACERDA EMA. Nutrition in obstetrics and paediatrics. Rio de Janeiro, p 369-392, 2009.

SCOTT JA; COBIAC L. The relationship between breastfeeding and weight status in a national sample of Australia children and adolescents. **Public Health**, p.1-6, 2012.

SIMON VG; SOUZA JMP; SOUZA SB. Breastfeeding, complementary feeding, overweight and obesity in preschool children. **Revista de Saúde Pública**. São Paulo, v.43 n.1, p.60-69, 2009.

VICTORA CG; MORRIS SS; BARROS FC; HORTA BL; WEIDERPASS E; TOMAS IE. Brestfeeding and growth in brazilian infants. **Am j clin nutr**, 1998.

VITOLO MR. Nutrition: from pregnancy to ageing. Rio de Janeiro, 2008.

TWELLS L; NEWHOOD KLN. Can exclusive breastfeeding reduce the lilelihood of childhood obesity in some region of Canada? **Canadian Journal Public Health**, v.101, p.36-39, 2012.

WHO. Protecting, promoting and supporting breast-feeding. Geneva: WHO; 1989.

WHO. The optimal duration of exclusive breastfeeding: report of an expert consultation, Geneva, 2001.

CHAPTER 12

RISK OF DEVELOPING DIABETES MELLITUS TYPE 2: a study of associated factors

José Auricélio Bernardo Cândido
Maria Irismar de Almeida
Francisco José Maia Pinto
Carlos Robson Bezerra de Medeiros
Rafaella Maria Monteiro Sampaio
Radmila Alves Alencar Viana
Maria Rosilene Cândido Moreira

INTRODUCTION

Diabetes mellitus (DM) is the term that describes a metabolic disorder of multiple etiology, characterised by chronic hyperglycaemia and disturbances in the metabolism of carbohydrates, lipids and proteins, resulting from defects in insulin secretion, insulin action or both (BRASIL, 2013).

There are two types of DM, with type 2 (DM2) being the most common, affecting over 90% of cases and characterised by defects in insulin action and secretion. It is estimated that approximately 347 million people worldwide have DM2 (DANAEI et al., 2011).

In Brazil, in 2012, the Ministry of Health estimated that there were more than 12 million diabetics in the country (BRASIL, 2016). A study on mortality from DM complications in Brazil found that the North and Northeast had the highest mortality rates. This demonstrates the existence of regional inequalities, since DM can be avoided mainly through preventive actions (KLAFKE et al., 2014).

Preventing or delaying the onset of diabetes through lifestyle modifications or pharmaceutical interventions has been demonstrated in randomised clinical trials in China, the United States, India and Organisation for Economic Co-operation and Development (OECD) countries, which has led several countries to implement diabetes prevention programmes. However, in order to reduce costs, individual intervention programmes are only aimed at individuals at high risk of developing the disease

(MENDES, 2011).

Although there is still no defined standardisation of risk factors for DM2, researchers on the subject say that the greater the number of risk factors present in each young person, the greater the chance of acquiring the disease (VASCONCELOS et al., 2010).

Thus, models and scores to predict the development of type 2 diabetes have been developed according to classic risk factors such as age, gender, obesity, metabolic factors, lifestyle, family history of diabetes and ethnicity. Examples include the American Diabetes Association's Diabetes Risk Test scale and the Finnish Diabetes Risk Score (FINDRISC) developed in Finland and validated in English (VALENTE; AZEVEDO, 2011).

Although the performance of these risk scores is far from desirable, in terms of public health, it is quite feasible, considering the low cost of this screening before carrying out laboratory screening with fasting blood glucose levels, the Oral Glucose Tolerance Test (OGTT) or the Glycated Haemoglobin Test (HbA1c) (LEITE; UMPIERREZ, 2015).

FINDRISC is a simple, fast, inexpensive and non-invasive method for determining the risk of developing DM2 over the next 10 years, as well as being able to identify individuals with undiagnosed diabetes and pre-diabetes (TANKOVA et al., 2011).

The search for early intervention in the risk factors for developing type 2 diabetes mellitus or slowing down its growth has been a concern for researchers all over the world. In order to understand, study and intervene in these risk factors, various studies have been carried out at national and international level and different instruments have been used to identify the prevalence of risk factors for DM2.

This study sought to analyse the risk of developing type 2 diabetes mellitus and associate it with sociodemographic, clinical and lifestyle variables, using the FINDRISC scale.

METHODS

This is a quantitative study with a descriptive and analytical approach, carried out in the District of Dourado, in the municipality of Horizonte-Ceará, between November 2015 and January 2016. The Dourado District was chosen for this study because it is the area with the largest number of registered families (5,527); it has the third largest population aged between 30 and 69; it has the largest number of people with diabetes registered (143) and monitored (137) at the Basic Health Unit (TABNET, 2015).

The study population was made up of individuals from the Dourado catchment area, in the municipality of Horizonte-Ceará, aged between 30 and 69, of both sexes. The study sample was calculated using the formula indicated for calculating cross-sectional studies with a finite population (SANTOS, 2015), resulting in 325 users, plus 10% for losses and/or dropouts, resulting in 358 participants.

The people to be surveyed were chosen from the **"A" forms of the Primary Care Information System (SIAB), which are** filled in by the Community Health Agents (ACS). Only the households and users of nine CHAs were listed, since one was on sick leave and was not monitoring his micro-area.

The numbers from the medical records were entered into IBM SSPS (Statistical Package for the Social Sciences) where a simple randomisation **of the cases** was carried out **("Random sample of cases") and the participants were chosen by** household and submitted to the questionnaires, in accordance with the inclusion and exclusion criteria. The study included people aged between 30 and 69, both sexes, accompanied by the CHA in their respective catchment area and who were at home at the time of the survey. Individuals with a previous diagnosis of type 1 or type 2 diabetes or any chronic condition that could directly interfere with anthropometric measurements were excluded from the study.

In cases where the chosen participants refused to answer the questionnaire (n=10) or were not at home at the time of the CHW's visit (n=06), new participants were sought, following the order in which the households were randomised, until the final sample number was reached; however, some CHWs, following the number of people in the age group of the families, administered a further 21 questionnaires, totalling 371 participants.

The outcome variable of this study was the risk of developing DM2 in 10 years and the explanatory variables were distributed into sociodemographic (gender and age), lifestyle (physical activity and fruit and vegetable intake) and clinical (weight, height, body mass index, waist circumference, use of antihypertensive medication, history of altered glucose and family history of DM2).

In order to identify individuals at high risk of progressing to diabetes and who could benefit from target prevention (primary prevention), the Finnish FINDRISK instrument was used, which determines the risk of developing the disease. The instrument consists of eight items that include information on age, blood pressure, body mass index (BMI), waist circumference (WC), physical activity, diet, use of antihypertensive medication, history of high blood glucose and family history of diabetes. The instrument used is quite feasible from the point of view of the public health actions in force in Brazil (BUIJSSE et al., 2011).

Risk was calculated based on the sum of the scores for each variable. The following risk scale was used: <7 points = low risk; 7 to 11 points = slightly high risk; 12 to 14 points = moderate risk; 15 to 20 points = high risk and >20 points = very high risk. In this study, low/moderate risk (<15) and high/very high risk (>15) were adopted (SALINERO-FORT et al., 2010; VALENTE; AZEVEDO, 2011).

To measure the subjects' weight, a Your Way portable digital scale with a capacity of 180 kg and an accuracy of 0.1 kg was used. To measure height and WC, a NYBC non-elastic tape measure with a length of 150 cm was used. The procedures for measuring weight, height and WC were standardised according to Brazil (2011).

After collecting weight and height data, the BMI of each interviewee was calculated, using the parameters of the World Health Organisation (1998) for classifying nutritional status. The parameters established by the World Health Organisation (1998) were also used to classify CHD risk.

The scores related to physical activity were weighted based on questions about whether the participants spent at least 30 minutes on it every day, either at work or during their free time.

With regard to the participants' diet, they were asked whether they ate fruit and vegetables daily or occasionally.

They were also asked about the occurrence of an elevated glucose level in any routine laboratory test or illness or during pregnancy. The heredity variable was approached by asking about kinship with people with DM2. Parents, siblings and children were given a higher score than first-degree relatives: cousins, uncles and grandparents.

The data was tabulated and double-entered into a Microsoft Excel spreadsheet and exported to the Statistical Package for Social Sciences (SPSS) software, version 18.0, for data processing.

The data was analysed descriptively using frequencies (absolute and percentage). Inferential statistics were used to compare the characteristics associated with the outcome, calculating prevalence ratios using Poisson regression at a significance level of 5%.

This study complied with the recommendations of Resolution 466/2012, **which regulates "research involving human beings" of the Council of the European Union.** National Health Programme. It was submitted to and approved by the Research Ethics Committee of the State University of Ceará (UECE), with CAAE opinion no. 47623615.6.0000.5534.

RESULTS

In this study, 371 people between the ages of 30 and 69 from the town of Dourado in the municipality of Horizonte, Ceará, took part.Among the prevalences found, the majority were: 317 (85.4%) for no/low/moderate risk of developing DM2 in ten years according to FINDRISK; 248 (66.8%) female; 218 (58.8%) were aged over 45; 270 (72.8%) high BMI; 292 (78.7%) increased WC; 201 (54.2%) practised physical activity; 249 (67.1%) did not eat vegetables and/or fruit regularly; 297 (80.1%) were not taking antihypertensive medication; 342 (92.2%) had no record of high blood glucose levels and 194 (52.3%) had a relative with type 1 or type 2 DM (Table 1).

Table 1: Characterisation of participants according to risk and sociodemographic, lifestyle and clinical variables in the district of Dourado, Horizonte, Ceará, 2016.

VARIABLES	N°	%
Risk of DM2		
< 15	317	85,4
> 15	54	14,6
Sex		
Male	123	33,2
Female	248	66,8
Age > 45 years		
Yes	218	58,8
No	153	41,2
Body Mass Index (BMI)		
Normal	101	27,2
Overweight / Obesity	270	72,8
Waist circumference (WC)		
Normal	79	21,3
Increased / Very Increased Risk	292	78,7
Physical activity		
Yes	201	54,2
No	170	45,8
Eat fruit/vegetables daily		
Yes	122	32,9
No	249	67,1

Taking antihypertensives		
Yes	74	19,9
No	297	80,1
History of impaired glucose		
Yes	29	07,8
No	342	92,2
Family history of DM2		
Yes	194	52,3
No	177	47,7

In relation to the participants who had a High/Very High risk of developing DM2 in ten years, it was found that the majority were female, **45 (18.1%); aged > 45 years, 35 (22.9%); who were obese (BMI > 30), 32 (26.7%); with increased WC,** 53 (18.2%); who didn't practice physical activity, 29 (17.1%); who didn't eat fruit/vegetables every day, 38 (15.3%); who took antihypertensive drugs, 32 (43.2%); who didn't have a history of altered glucose, 37 (10.8%) and people with a family history of DM2, 51 (26.3%) (Table 2).

Among the variables analysed, the risk of developing DM2 in ten years was statistically significant at the 5% level for gender ($p=0.005$) and age ($p<0.001$) and highly significant for the clinical variables BMI ($p<0.001$), WC ($p<0.001$) use of antihypertensive drugs ($p<0.001$), altered glucose test ($p<0.001$) and heredity ($p<0.001$). There was no statistically significant association with physical activity ($p=0.209$) and eating fruit and vegetables daily ($p=0.582$).

Table 2: Association between the risk of developing DM2 in ten years and sociodemographic, clinical and lifestyle variables in the district of Dourado, Horizonte, Ceará, 2015.

VARIABLES		Total	DM2 RISK CLASSIFICATION				P*
			High/ Very high		**None Low/Moderate**		
			N	**%**	**N**	**%**	
Sex							
	Female	248	45	18,1	203	81,9	**0,005**
	Male	123	9	7,3	114	92,7	
Age £ 45							
	Yes	218	35	22,9	118	77,1	**< 0,001**
	No	153	19	8,7	199	91,3	
BMI							
	Normal < 30	251	22	8,8	229	91,2	**< 0,001**
	Obesity > 30	120	32	26,7	88	73,3	
Waist circumference (WC)							
	Increased	292	53	18,2	239	81,8	**< 0,001**
	Not Increased	79	1	1,3	78	98,7	
Physical activity							
	Yes	201	25	12,4	176	87,6	0,209

No	170	29	17,1	141	82,9	
Eat fruit/vegetables daily						
Every day	122	16	13,1	106	86,9	0,582
Not every day	249	38	15,3	211	84,7	
Taking antihypertensives						
Yes	74	32	43,2	42	56,8	**< 0,001**
No	297	22	7,4	275	92,6	
History of impaired glucose						
Yes	29	17	58,6	12	41,4	**< 0,001**
No	342	37	10,8	305	89,2	
Family history of DM2						
Yes	194	51	26,3	143	73,7	**< 0,001**
No	177	3	1,7	174	98,3	

DISCUSSION

The high risk of developing DM2 presupposes conditions in which the individual has not yet reached the level of pre-diabetes (a situation in which blood glucose is above normal, but not yet diagnosed with diabetes). Thus, people at high risk of DM2 are more likely to develop the disease (MARINHO, 2010). In this case, screening is recommended with the aim of finding out the person's previous history; carrying out a physical examination, including checking blood pressure, anthropometric data (weight, height and WC) and calculating BMI; identifying risk factors for DM; assessing health conditions and requesting the necessary laboratory tests that can contribute to the diagnosis and therapeutic or preventive decision (BRASIL, 2013). In view of this, sociodemographic, clinical and lifestyle factors were identified as variables in this study for screening people at risk of developing DM2 in ten years, based on the FINDRISK questionnaire.

In relation to the demographic variable gender, this study shows that the majority were female and the risk of developing DM2 in ten years was high/very high. These data were similar to those found in the literature (PETERMANN et al., 2015). Another study showed an approximate parity between the sexes (MEDEIROS et al., 2012). Thus, it can be seen that there is still no consensus in the studies researched on the prevalence of DM2 in relation to gender.

Some authors have tried to explain the majority findings for females in their research, suggesting that women's participation in research is due to the fact that they are more concerned about their health than men, and that men have a deficit in self-care (FONTES et al., 2011; PETERMANN et al., 2015). It is therefore understood that more in-depth and comparable quantitative studies are needed to show statistical significance in relation to gender when associated with risk factors for DM2.

Among the participants in this study, 14.6% had a high or very high risk of developing DM2 in the next 10 years. These results are different to those found in other studies carried out around the world, as cited in the literature: 19.5 per cent in Spain (DIABETES FOUNDATION, 2011); 12.8 per cent in Portugal (SARTORELLI et al., 2006; VALENTE and AZEVEDO, 2012); 10.5 per cent in Cuba (NARANJO et al., 2013) and 28.5 per cent in Norway (HJELLSET et al., 2011).

In Brazil, a prevalence of 27 per cent was found in Colantina-ES (BRUNO et al., 2014); the lowest prevalence was found in the municipality of Tubarão-SC (3.8 per cent) (BITTENCOURT; VINHOLES, 2013). In the Northeast, studies were found in Campina Grande-PB (MEDEIROS et al., 2012) and Picos-PI (BARROS et al., 2014); however, these studies did not report a high risk of DM2. In Ceará, Marinho et al. (2013), in a similar study, identified 11.7% in the municipality of Itapipoca. In Fortaleza, studies by Macedo et al. (2010) and Lima et al. (2014) investigated risk factors but did not determine the prevalence of high/very high risk of developing DM2 over ten years.

In view of the values, it is assumed that there is no set percentage for calculating the high/very high risk of developing DM2 in ten years, since this value is directly related to the population studied and their risk factors.

Checking for an association between the risk of developing DM2 in ten years and sociodemographic and clinical variables, statistical significance was observed, suggesting that these factors are present in people at high/very high risk of DM2.

Statistical significance was also found for the same variables in studies carried out in Campina Grande-PB (MEDEIROS et al., 2012) and in Itapipoca and Fortaleza, Ceará (MARINHO et al., 2012; LIMA et al., 2014). Other authors have also investigated the same risk factors for DM2, showing their prevalence and statistical significance (BARROS et al., 2014; BRUNO et al., 2014; FLOR et al., 2015; ZARDO et al., 2015).

With regard to clinical anthropometric variables, BMI values indicate that most of the interviewees are overweight and obese, while WC values show that most of the interviewees are at very high risk of metabolic diseases.

The high prevalence of overweight individuals with DM and/or a predominance of increased WC was found in other epidemiological studies (SALINERO-FORT et al., 2010; VASCONCELOS et al., 2010; MEDEIROS et al., 2012; VALENTE and AZEVEDO, 2012; FLOR et al., 2015). Thus, it can be seen that there is an association between physical activity and the quality of the diet, which affects anthropometric measurements and, consequently, the risk of developing DM2.

CONCLUSION

It was concluded that, based on the FINDRISK questionnaire, the factors associated with the risk of developing diabetes were: age > 45 years, BMI > 30, increased WC, inadequate physical activity, inadequate fruit and/or vegetable intake, use of antihypertensive drugs, history of altered glucose levels and history of DM in 1st and/or 2nd degree relatives. With regard to modifiable factors for DM2, this study identified a high prevalence of central obesity, overweight/obesity and inadequate diet.

When relating risk to sociodemographic, clinical and lifestyle factors, it was noted that the sociodemographic variables (gender and age) were statistically significant ($p < 0.005$) in relation to DM2. In relation to the clinical variables (BMI, WC, altered glucose, use of antihypertensive drugs and heredity), all showed statistical significance in relation to the disease.

The lifestyle variables (physical activity and eating fruit and vegetables daily) did not show direct statistical significance with DM2, but these practices did influence the values of the clinical variables.

A possible limitation of the questionnaire is that the intensity of physical activity was not identified, nor were the habits of eating fruit and vegetables made clear, which could be a bias in the results of future research in terms of statistical significance. Thus, this study helped to identify not only the number of participants, but also those who were at high/very high risk of developing DM2, as well as the associated factors.

It is hoped that this study can contribute to the adoption of preventive measures through therapeutic plans accompanied by multi-professional teams that raise awareness of risk factors, lifestyle changes and healthy habits, improving health, quality of life and changing the high risk score level to the moderate or low risk level of developing diabetes mellitus.

REFERENCES

BARROS KCS, LIMA MA, SILVA ARV, ALMEIDA PC, MACHADO ALG. Risk factors for type 2 diabetes mellitus in employees of a public university. **Revista de**

Enfermagem UFPE on line, v.8, n.9, p.3099- 105, 2014.

BITTENCOURT A, VINHOLES DB. Estimating the risk of type 2 diabetes mellitus in bank employees in the city of Tubarão, state of Santa Catarina, Brazil. **Scientia Medica**, v.23, n.2, p.82-9, 2013.

BRAZIL. Ministry of Health. Health Care Secretariat. Department of Primary Care. Guidelines for collecting and analysing anthropometric data in health services: Technical Standard for the Food and Nutrition Surveillance System - SISVAN. Brasília, 2011. 76p.

BRAZIL. Ministry of Health. Health Care Secretariat. Department of Primary Care. Strategies for the care of people with chronic diseases: Diabetes Mellitus. Brasília, DF: Ministry of Health, 2013. 160p. (Primary Care Notebooks, n. 36).

BRAZIL. Ministry of Health. Indicators and Data from Brazil - IDB - 2012. Indicators of risk and protective factors. Prevalence of diabetes mellitus. Brasília DF. 2016.

BRUNO A, PEREIRA LR, ALMEIDA HS. Assessment of the prevalence of risk factors for the development of type 2 diabetes mellitus in patients at the Unesc Health Clinic. Espírito Santo. **Demetra: Food, Nutrition & Health**, v.9, n.3, p.661-680, 2014.

BUIJSSE B, SIMMONS RK, GRIFFIN SJ, SCHULZE MB. Risk Assessment Tools For Identifying Individuals at Risk of Developing Type 2 Diabetes. **Revista de Epidemiologia**, v.33, n.1, p.46-62, 2011.

DANAEI, G.; FINUCANE, M.M.; LU, Y.; SINGH, G.M.; COWAN, M.J.; PACIOREK, C.J.; et al. National, regional, and global trends in fasting plasma glucose and diabetes prevalence since 1980: systematic analysis of health examination surveys and epidemiological studies with 370 country-years and *2-7* million participants. **Lancet**, v.378, n.9785, 31-40, 2011.

DIABETES FOUNDATION. Microvascular and macrovascular complications of diabetes. **Clinicai Diabetes Journals**, v.29, p.116-22, 2011.

FLOR LS, CAMPOS MR, OLIVEIRA AF, SCHRAMM JMA. Diabetes burden in Brazil: fraction attributable to overweight, obesity and excess weight. **Revista de Saúde Pública**, v.49, n.29, p.1-11, 2015.

FONTES WD, BARBOZA TM, LEITE MC, FONSECA RLS, SANTOS LCF, NERY TCL. Men's health care: dialogue between teaching and service. **Acta Paulista de Enfermagem**, v.24, n.3, p.430-3, 2011.

HJELLSET VT, BJORGE B, ERIKSEN HR, HOSTMARK AT. Risk Factors for Type 2 Diabetes Among Female Pakistani Immigrants: The InvaDiab-DEPLAN Study on Pakistani Immigrant Women Living in Oslo, Norway. J. **Immigrant Minority Health**, v.13, n.1, p.101-10, 2011.

KLAFKE A, DUNCANET BB, ROSA RS, MOURA L, MALTA DC, SCHMIDT MI. Mortality due to acute complications of diabetes mellitus in Brazil, 20062010. **Epidemiologia e Serviços de Saúde**, v.23, n.3, p.455-462, 2014.

LEITE SAO, UMPIERREZ G. Primary prevention of type 2 diabetes: how to translate the results of clinical studies for application in public health. In: Diabetes in Clinical Practice, Brazilian Diabetes Society, e-book 2.0, mod. 3, chap.3, 2015. Available at: http://ebook.diabetes.org.br/.

LIMA ACS, ARAÚJO MFM, FREITAS RWJF, ZANETTI ML, ALMEIDA PC, DAMASCENO MMC. Risk factors for type 2 diabetes mellitus in university students: association with sociodemographic variables. **Revista Latino- Americana de Enfermagem**, v.22, n.3, p.484-90, 2014.

MACEDO SF, ARAÚJO MFM, MARINHO NPB, LIMA ACS, FREITAS RWF, DAMASCENO MMC. Risk factors for type 2 diabetes mellitus in children. **Revista Latino-Americana de Enfermagem**, v.18, n.5, 2010.

MARINHO NBP. Risk Assessment for Type 2 Diabetes Mellitus among adults in Itapipoca - Ceará, 2010, 90p, Dissertation (master's degree), UFC, Fortaleza, CE.

MARINHO NBP, VASCONCELOS HCA, ALENCAR AMPG, ALMEIDA PC, DAMASCENO MMC. Diabetes mellitus: associated factors among users of the family health strategy. **Acta Paulista de Enfermagem**, v.25, n.4, p.595- 600, 2012.

MARINHO NBP, VASCONCELOS HCA, ALENCAR AMPG, ALMEIDA PC, DAMASCENO MMC. Risk of type 2 diabetes mellitus and associated factors. **Acta Paulista de Enfermagem**, v.26, n.6, p.569-74, 2013.

MEDEIROS CCM, BESSA GG, COURA AS, FRANÇA ISX, SOUSA FS. Prevalence of risk factors for diabetes mellitus among civil servants. **Revista Eletrônica de Enfermagem**, v.14, n.3, p.559-69, 2012.

MENDES EV. Health care networks. Brasília: Pan American Health Organisation, 2011. 549 p.

NARANJO AA, RODRÍGUEZ ÁY, LLERA RE, AROCHE R. Diabetes risk in a Cuban primary care setting in persons with no known glucose abnormalities. **Medicc Rev**, v.15, n.2, p.16-9, 2013.

PETERMANN XB, MACHADO IS, PIMENTEL BN, MIOLO SB, MARTINS LR, FEDOSSE E. Epidemiology and care of Diabetes Mellitus practised in Primary Health Care: a narrative review. **Revista Saúde**, v.41, n.1, p.49-56, 2015.

SALINERO-FORT MA, PAU ECS, ABÁNADES-HERRANZ JC, DUJOVNE-KOHAN I, CÁRDENAS-VALLADOLID J. Baseline risk of diabetes mellitus in primary care according to the FINDRISC questionnaire, associated factors and clinical evolution after 18 months of follow-up. **Revista Clinica Española**, v.210, n.9, p.448-53, 2010.

SANTOS GEO. Sample calculation: online calculator. Available at: <http://www.calculoamostral.vai.la>.

SARTORELLI D S, FRANCO LJ, CARDOSO MA. Nutritional intervention and primary prevention of type 2 diabetes mellitus: a systematic review.

Cadernos de Saúde Publica, v.22, n.1, p.7-18, 2006.

TABNET. Ministry of Health. DATASUS. Information Technology at the Service of the SUS. Primary Care Attention System, SIAB. 2015.

TANKOVA T, CHAKAROVA N, ATANASSOVA I, DAKOVSKA L. Evaluation of the Finnish Diabetes Risk Score as a screening tool for impaired fasting glucose, impaired glucose tolerance and undetected diabetes. **Diabetes Research and Clinical Practice**, v.92, n.1, p.46-52, 2011.

VALENTE T, AZEVEDO L. RADAR Study: Increased Risk of Diabetes in Amarante. **Revista Portuguesa de Medicina Geral e Familiar**, v.28, n.1, p.18- 24, 2012.

VASCONCELOS HCA, ARAÚJO MFM, DAMASCENO MMC, ALMEIDA PC, FREITAS RWJF. Risk factors for type 2 diabetes mellitus among adolescents. **Revista de Escola de Enfermagem**, v.44, n.4, p.881-7, 2010.

WORLD HEALTH ORGANISATION. Heart Promotion Glossary. Geneva: WHO, 1998.

ZARDO M, BASSAN MB, FARIAS KCM, DIEFENTHAELER HS, GRAZZIOTIN NA. Tracking risk factors for type 2 diabetes in workers of an industry from the city of Concordia-SC. **Perspectiva, Erechim**, v.39, n.145, p.85-95, 2015.

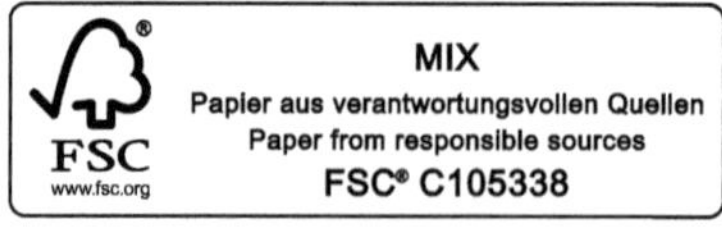

Printed by Books on Demand GmbH, Norderstedt / Germany